## Other Titles in THE **COMPLETE GUIDE** SERIES

The Complete Guide to
Circuit Training
by Debbie Lawrence, Bob Hope

The Complete Guide to
Postnatal Fitness
by Judy DiFiore

Complete Guide to
Endurance Training
by Jon Ackland

The Complete Guide to
Strength Training
by Anita Bean

The Complete Guide to
Exercise in Water
by Debbie Lawrence

The Complete Guide to
Stretching
by Christopher Norris

The Complete Guide to
Core Stability
by Matt Lawrence

The Complete Guide to
Sports Massage
by Tim Paine

THE COMPLETE GUIDE TO

Debbie Lawrence

# EXERCISE TO MUSIC

2nd edition

A & C Black • London

**Note**

Whilst every effort has been made to ensure that the content of this book is as technically accurate and as sound as possible, neither the editors nor the publishers can accept responsibility for any injury or loss sustained as a result of the use of this material

First published 1999 by
A & C Black Ltd
37 Soho Square, London W1D 3QZ
www.acblack.com

Second edition 2004
First edition 1999

ISBN 0 7136 6778 8

A CIP catalogue record for this book is available from the British Library

**Acknowledgements**
Cover photography © Corbis
Line illustrations © Jean Ashley

A & C Black uses paper produced with elemental chlorine-free pulp, harvested from managed sustainable forests.

Typeset in 10½ on 12pt Baskerville BE Regular

Printed and bound in Great Britain by
Biddles Ltd, Kings Lynn.

# CONTENTS

# ACKNOWLEDGEMENTS

There are many people who I need to thank, for their help, support and encouragement:

The late Lesley Mowbray of Central YMCA for commissioning me to write this book and also for providing me with the opportunity to work with a team of multi-talented fitness professionals who are all truly committed to the promotion of health-related exercise.

All my colleagues at YMCA Fitness Industry Training – you are truly a professional, dedicated and inspirational team. It is a pleasure to work with and know you all. With special thanks to Alex Carr for contributing her choreography ideas.

Mary Lawrence for encouraging me to work in the fitness industry.

Roy Lawrence – thanks.

Jamie Lawrence – my brother and my friend.

Jane Fonda, whose videos inspired me and many others to teach.

Dorothy Scopes of The Keep Fit Association, with whom I began my teacher training.

Everyone who has ever participated in my exercise classes, Fiona O'Neill, Karen Wright, Alison MaCall, Therese and Farideh.

To the many teachers I have trained over the years – I have learned masses from you all and it is lovely for me to see you all achieving success in the industry.

Gabby Groves of the Exercise Association of England for introducing me to Jonathan Taylor of A & C Black.

Hannah McEwen and Charlotte Jenkins at A & C Black for working with me on the 2nd edition. Thanks for your encouragement and positive support.

# INTRODUCTION

Dancing and movement to music have been popular recreational activities for centuries. By comparison, exercising to music is a relatively new leisure pursuit. One of the first organisations to provide movement and fitness classes using music was The Keep Fit Association of England. These movement-based classes to music were designed to promote activity and provide a social environment primarily for women to exercise and enjoy themselves.

The more recent 'aerobics' boom of the early 1980s developed yet another alternative approach to exercising to music, and has proven to be the greatest influence on the evolution of exercise to music (ETM) sessions as we know them today. Indeed, over the last decade a whole variety of ETM programmes have been developed, including step, slide, new body, cardio funk, sculpt, supple strength, core ball and spinning. It is interesting to note that despite the introduction of these very diverse approaches to ETM, many people still consider exercise to music to be a dance-based activity!?

The aim of this book is to explore the benefits of ETM regardless of its different guises.

**Section 1** explores the components of fitness and how they can be improved. It also explores the advantages and disadvantages of exercising to music; the different ways music can be used in a session and choreography tools.

**Section 2** outlines the safety considerations when exercising to music and explores a variety of different programme formats. It explains and illustrates appropriate activities for warming up and cooling down in an ETM session.

**Section 3** explores different approaches to cardio-vascular, muscular strength and endurance, and flexibility training to music. It explains how each component of an ETM session should be structured and illustrates a range of different exercises that can be used to develop different ETM programmes. It also introduces sessions that incorporate a 'mind and body' feel. Providing basic exercises from pilates and yoga.

This second edition also provides example lesson plans.

# WHY EXERCISE TO MUSIC?

PART **ONE**

# THE BENEFITS OF EXERCISE TO MUSIC

## What are the general benefits of exercise to music?

Exercise to music (ETM) is a safe and effective method of exercising that is enjoyed by a variety of people. A well-designed ETM programme can improve all the components of fitness that contribute to the physical fitness of an individual. The most essential components for maintaining our fitness for life, and fitness to participate in sporting activities are: cardio-vascular fitness, muscular strength, muscular endurance, and flexibility. Sportspeople, however, also need training in specific skill-related components, referred to as motor fitness. These skill-related components include: agility, balance, reaction time, speed, power and co-ordination.

Being physically fit also contributes to our overall health, or total fitness. Total fitness includes social, mental, emotional, nutritional and medical fitness. This chapter explores and discusses each of the components of physical and total fitness. It also identifies how exercise to music can improve our physical fitness and lead to total fitness.

## What is cardio-vascular fitness?

Cardio-vascular fitness is the ability of the heart, lungs and circulatory system to transport and utilise oxygen efficiently. It is sometimes referred to as cardio-respiratory fitness, stamina, or aerobic fitness.

## Why do we need cardio-vascular fitness?

A strong heart and efficient respiratory and circulatory system are essential for maintaining our quality of life; they are also essential to enable us to safely participate in sporting and recreational activities. A weak heart and inefficient respiratory and circulatory system are more susceptible to diseases that cause premature death. Indeed, coronary heart disease is the highest cause of death in the Western world. Increased physical activity and improved cardio-vascular fitness can help prevent cardio-vascular diseases.

In the long-term, specific training to improve cardio-vascular fitness will improve the efficiency of the heart, lungs and blood vessels. The heart becomes stronger, allowing it to pump a greater volume of blood in each contraction (stroke volume); the capillary network in our muscles expands, allowing the transportation of more oxygen to the body cells and the swifter removal of waste products; and the size and number of mitochondria, the cells in which aerobic energy is produced, increases, which, in turn, enables us to deliver and utilise the oxygen that our muscles receive more effectively. Since oxygen is essential for our long-term production of energy, our ability to perform aerobic activities will improve. This will enable us to perform such activities for a longer period of time.

Activities which make demands on the cardio-vascular system increase the metabolic rate, i.e. the rate at which we use energy or burn calories. Therefore, frequent performance of these activities will assist with the reduction of body fat and the lowering of cholesterol levels, which will assist with effective weight management. The increased strength and efficiency of the cardio-vascular system, coupled with the reduction in body fat and cholesterol levels may also potentially contribute to the normalising of elevated blood pressure, all of which have a positive effect on our health.

## Summary of the long-term benefits of cardio-vascular training

- Stronger heart muscle.
- Increased stroke volume (amount of blood pumped in each contraction of the heart).
- Increased capillarisation (more blood vessels delivering blood and oxygen to the muscles).
- Increased mitochrondria (cells in which aerobic energy is produced).
- Inceased metabolic rate (rate at which we burn calories).
- Decreased body fat.
- Decreased cholesterol levels.
- Decreased blood pressure.
- Decreased risk of coronary heart disease.

## How can we improve our cardio-vascular fitness?

To improve the fitness of the heart, respiratory and circulatory system we need to perform rhythmic activities which use the large muscles of the body. These should be performed on a regular basis, ideally between three to five times per week, and at a moderate intensity to create a feeling of mild breathlessness, without any unnecessary discomfort; we should be able to comfortably sustain these activities for a prolonged duration. Traditional activities that promote this type of fitness are walking, running, cycling, aerobic dancing, rowing and swimming etc. Adherence to this type of exercise programme will induce the necessary long-term health-related improvements to the cardio-vascular system. The recommended training requirements for improving cardio-vascular fitness are outlined in table 1.1.

## How can we improve our cardio-vascular fitness in an ETM programme

The traditional activities that improve cardio-vascular fitness are running, cycling, walking, swimming and rowing. Each of these activities utilises the larger muscles of the body and requires the body weight to be locomoted against a resistance. Walking, running and cycling require greater use of the lower body and minimal work of the upper body; they require the body to move against the force of gravity. Alternatively, swimming and rowing require the muscles of the upper body to have a much greater involvement; they require the body to be moved against the resistance of the water.

The most effective types of exercises to bring about the desired training benefits and improve cardio-vascular fitness in an ETM session are those that require us to use the large muscles of the lower body to move our body weight against the force of gravity. Movements which require us to jump up, bend deeply and travel are very effective. These are illustrated in figure 1.1 (*see* page 4).

Jumping, leaping and explosive movements require plenty of muscular effort to move our centre of gravity away from the ground. As our body travels back down to the floor we pick up greater momentum, so to land safely we need our muscles to work harder to maintain correct alignment of the joints. If excessive jumping

| Table 1.1 | The recommended training requirements for improving cardio-vascular fitness |
|---|---|
| **Frequency** How often should we perform these activities | Between three to five times a week, ideally varying the activities we perform and altering the impact to avoid repetitive strain or injury to the muscles and joints. |
| **Intensity** How hard should we be working? | At an intensity which causes the pulse rate to increase to somewhere between 55% and 90% of its maximum is sufficient. Lower levels of intensity are appropriate for less active populations. |
| **Time** How long should we sustain these activities for? | Between 15 and 60 minutes is an optimal duration, with approximately 20 minutes sufficient to mantain fitness. less fit groups may need to progress gradually to this duration. |
| **Type** What types of activities are most effective? | Activities which are rhythmic, use the large muscles, and are aerobic (require oxygen) in nature. For example, swimming, running, or cycling. |

(high-impact) movements are used, however, greater stress will be placed on the joints, so they should be combined with other lower impact activities to avoid causing injury.

Since travelling movements require us to shift the resistance of our body across the force of gravity, we need to exert greater muscular effort and utilise a larger number of muscles to create such movements. Travelling movements which require us to move in many different directions, are excellent for varying the stress placed on the weight-bearing joints. An ETM programme which utilises a variety of travelling movements is potentially much safer and far less stressful on the body than one which uses exercises performed in the same position, such as jogging and jumping on the spot.

Deep bending movements such as squats and lunges are also very effective. These exercises utilise the large muscles of the legs to contract, bending and straightening the knee and hip joints, and transferring the weight of our body against the force of gravity. These movements are very effective, but if too many bending movements occur, there will be greater likelihood of repetitive strain to the moving joints. It is, therefore, advisable to combine a mixture of jumping, bending and travelling movements to promote a safer and less stressful programme.

Movements that utilise the muscles of the upper body are comparatively less effective in

**Figure 1.1 Movement of the centre of gravity during jumping, bending and travelling movements: (a) jogging on the spot or jumping movements lift the weight of the body and the centre of gravity upwards through a large range of motion; (b) travelling movements (i.e. walking) involves the work of more muscles and increases the range of motion by moving the centre of the body across the force of gravity; (c) squatting or bending requires the body weight and centre of gravity to be shifted downwards and then upwards against the force of gravity**

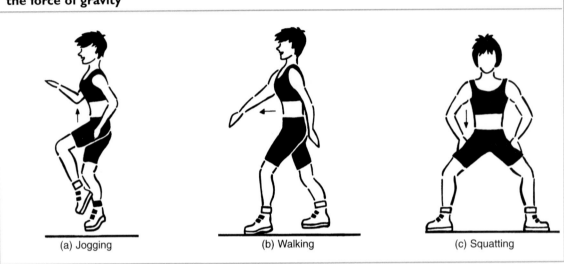

(a) Jogging      (b) Walking      (c) Squatting

improving cardio-vascular fitness because the muscles primarily responsible for performing such movements (deltoids, biceps, trapezius etc.) are smaller than the large leg muscles. Also, the resistance they are moving (the arms) is relatively insignificant in producing a demand for oxygen. Movement of the arms above the head will elevate the heart rate due to the heart having to work harder to pump blood upwards against the force of gravity. Continuous arm work above the head, however, may have an adverse effect on blood pressure, which is neither desirable nor recommended. Therefore, while the arms can be used with the legs to add variety to choreography, it is essential that the emphasis is on leg movements to ensure the programme is effective.

## How can we cater for different fitness levels?

The intensity of activities selected should correspond to the fitness level of participants. The activities selected for a less fit person need to be of a low intensity because their heart will have to work harder to deliver the same volume of blood, and their muscles will be less efficient at making effective use of the oxygen they receive. Therefore, very intense movements such as Jumping Jacks and Deep Squats should be adapted to make them less intense. This can be achieved by using slightly slower movements, bending the legs less deeply, taking out jumps (lowering impact) and by travelling less. Low-impact (those which involve no jumping) exercises are generally safer for a less fit group; higher impact exercises require a greater body awareness and strong muscular fixation for them to be performed effectively and for safe alignment to be maintained. Low-impact exercises are generally less stressful for the joints and can be less intense making them easier to perform correctly with safe alignment.

Fitter participants will need to be challenged; their heart will be strong and able to supply oxygen with less effort, and their muscles will make more effective use of the oxygen delivered. Therefore, they should be encouraged to put greater effort into all of their movements and can be encouraged to bend deeper, jump higher and travel more frequently during the programme. They can also be encouraged to move at a faster pace and perform explosive power moves (slower and stronger moves) more regularly throughout the programme. It is also safer for them to perform a large proportion of higher impact moves because their body awareness and skill levels are, or should be, greater and their muscles stronger. Both these factors promote the maintenance of correct alignment and form, which will enhance the safety of any exercise.

## What is flexibility?

Flexibility is the ability of our joints and muscles to move through their full potential range of motion. It is sometimes referred to as suppleness or mobility.

## Why do we need flexibility?

The ability of the joints and muscles to move through their full potential range of motion is essential for easing the performance of all of our everyday tasks. We need flexibility in our shoulder joints to reach our arms above our head when we change a light bulb, or reach for an object on a high shelf; we need flexibility in our hip joints to lift up our knees to climb stairs,

and to take long strides when walking. If we are flexible, we can move more efficiently.

Flexible joints and muscles also contribute to the maintenance of correct posture and joint alignment. Improved posture can potentially enhance our physical appearance, indeed, standing tall and upright can have a slimming effect on most body frames. Being sufficiently flexible will allow us to move with greater ease, and with greater poise.

On the other hand, a lack of flexibility will cause our bodies to become stiff and immobile; we will be less able to reach up to a high shelf, and less able to bend down to tie our shoe laces. This can restrict the everyday movements we are able to perform, and make us less self-sufficient. Moving around with an incorrect posture and joint alignment will potentially create muscle imbalance and increase our risk of injury. Poor posture will also create a less aesthetically pleasing appearance. Therefore, being flexible is of paramount importance for improving the quality and economy of our movements in everyday life.

Being sufficiently flexible will also contribute to the enhancement of our performance during sporting and recreational activities. If we are not sufficiently flexible we are more susceptible to injury when performing sporting activities, especially those that require us to move quickly into extended positions, such as bending down, reaching up and away, and twisting around. Some sporting activities, however, require much more flexibility than we need to perform our daily tasks, particularly some martial arts and dance activities, which require excessive flexibility. If we are too flexible, and the muscles and ligaments around the joint are not strong enough to keep the joint stable, there is a risk of injury.

Ultimately, we need the right amount of flexibility to perform our everyday tasks and to maintain correct alignment, but if we partici-pate in sporting activities we may require a little extra. A competitive sportsperson or professional dancer will need greater flexibility to assist with the achievement of their goals. However, if we participate in sporting activities for recreational purposes we must consider how far we should push ourselves. The key issue is to decide on the reasons for participating and the individual's aims. Ideally, we should ensure that we are flexible enough to meet the demands placed on our body without placing our bodies at risk from injury.

---

## Summary of the long-term benefits of flexibility training

- Improved range of motion in the joints and muscles.
- Improved posture and joint alignment.
- Enhanced performance of sporting and everyday activities.
- Reduced tension in the muscles.
- Reduced risk of injury when moving into extended positions.

---

## How can we improve flexibility?

Flexibility can be maintained by the frequent (daily) performance of activities that require our muscles and joints to move through their full range of motion. Since most lifestyles do not naturally provide these opportunities, stretching exercises are incorporated into most fitness programmes. Stretching exercises are those which require the two ends of the muscle, the origin and insertion, to move further apart. This causes the muscle to lengthen, and will potentially increase the range of motion at the joint. However, the muscle must also be allowed to relax to achieve an effective stretch.

**Static stretch positions** are generally advocated as safer. These stretches use comfortable, supportive positions which are held for an appropriate duration. They enable the tension initially felt in the muscle (the stretch reflex) to dissipate (desensitisation) which allows the muscle to relax and move safely to an extended range of movement. Stretching in this way can potentially improve our flexibility. If, however, we move too quickly or too far into the stretch (overstretching), then relaxation (desensitisation) of the muscle may not occur. It is therefore essential that we listen carefully to our body, and move only to the point of mild tension.

**Ballistic movements** which require the body to move quickly into an extended range of motion are not recommended. They can prevent desensitisation occurring and may potentially create muscle tearing and damage to the ligaments and other tissues which surround the joint. In the long term ballistic stretching may reduce the stability of the joints causing hypermobility (laxity or looseness of the ligaments around the joints), or cause irreparable damage to the muscles and joints, which may ultimately reduce the range of motion and decrease flexibility. Therefore, while some sporting activities still include ballistic stretching as part of their training, static stretches are more appropriate for the general population.

**Range of motion stretches** which involve lengthening the muscle at a controlled speed through the full range of motion can be used, although it could be argued that they do not allow sufficient time for the stretch reflex to desensitise. This would, to some extent, depend on the flexibility of the person and the speed at which the movement is performed. Care must be taken not to move too quickly or too far into the stretch otherwise the stretch may become ballistic in nature and may potentially cause injury. Range of motion stretches are only recommended for individuals with good flexibility and body awareness. The recommended training requirements for improving flexibility are outlined in table 1.2.

| **Table 1.2** | **The recommended training requirements for improving flexibility** |
|---|---|
| *Frequency*<br>How often should we perform these activities | Every day. The body must be warm prior to stretching to prevent muscle tearing and to enhance the range of motion achieved. |
| *Intensity*<br>How hard should we be working? | The positions selected should allow the muscle to lengthen and relax and achieve a slightly greater range of motion than normal. |
| *Time*<br>How long should we sustain these activities for? | Stretches can be held for approximately 8 to 30 seconds. For improvements in flexibility longer durations are necessary, but the body must be warm and relaxed. |
| *Type*<br>What types of activities are most effective? | Positions which allow one muscle to lengthen and relax while the opposing muscle is relaxed (passive static stretches) are most effective for improving flexibilty. |

## How can we improve our flexibility in an ETM programme?

It is important to stretch the muscles at the end of the warm-up to prepare them for the main workout; it is also important to stretch the muscles after the main workout to maintain their range of motion. The reasons for stretching at different points in the session will be discussed in greater depth in later chapters, which explore appropriate activities for warming up and cooling down.

There are two types of stretches which may be used in an ETM session: static stretches and range of motion (moving) stretches. To improve flexibility, static developmental stretches must be included in the programme. These stretches involve the muscle being lengthened to the end of the range of motion, where a mild tension is felt (stretch reflex). When the tension in the muscle eases (desensitises), the stretch can then be taken further. At this point the tension will reoccur in the muscle to prevent overstretching. The tension should be allowed to ease off, and when it does the stretch can be held for longer. This process can be repeated a number of times, if desired. Once an appropriate and extended range of motion is achieved, the stretch should be held for as long as is comfortable. However, in an ETM session time may be limited (depending on the nature of the session). If so, holding the stretch for about 30 seconds should be sufficient to bring about improvements in flexibility. Static stretching should be performed daily to bring about the desired results more rapidly and should only be performed when the muscles are very warm. It is recommended that within an ETM session they are included at the end of the class when the muscles have finished working; it is not effective to include this type of stretching after the warm-up and before the main workout. First, the muscles are probably not as warm as they need to be; second, the muscles will be working throughout the main session and therefore any improvements made will be wasted.

Moving stretches are those which require the muscle to lengthen slowly to the end of the range of motion, again to the point of a mild tension, but instead of holding the stretch in the extended position you move slowly out of the stretch and back to the start position. This process can be repeated a number of times, progressively and steadily moving into and out of the stretch position. It is worth noting that great care should be taken when performing moving stretches. If they are performed too quickly, the end of the range of motion may be reached too soon causing the muscle to contract to prevent damage occurring to the muscle or joint (a ballistic stretch). They should therefore only be used by experienced exercisers who are able to control their movements, and individuals who are able to recognise the body signals that indicate they are stretching too far.

## How can we cater for different levels of flexibility?

Less flexible participants will generally need to work through a small range of motion. Static stretches will be easiest for them to perform and will allow them to control the range of motion they work through. It should be easier for their muscles to relax if the stretch is held still. It may also be necessary to adapt some stretch positions for less flexible participants. Positions which assist balance (using a wall or floor-based positions) should allow them to stretch more comfortably; isolating stretches and using easier positions are also more appropriate.

More flexible participants should be able to move quite safely through a larger range of motion. They should be encouraged to fully extend (straighten) their joints, without locking them (hyperextending) and to move to their full potential. Combination stretches, where two muscles are stretched at the same time, are acceptable, since they should have sufficient body awareness to achieve an effective stretch of both muscles. Moving stretches are also safer when dealing with more flexible participants, provided they have sufficient body awareness and muscular control of their movements.

## What is muscular strength and endurance?

Muscular strength is the ability of our muscles to exert a near maximal force to lift a resistance. Muscular endurance is the ability of our muscles to continue contracting against a resistance.

## Why do we need muscular strength and endurance?

Our muscles need to be strong enough and have sufficient endurance to carry out daily tasks which require us to lift, carry, pull or push a resistance. This may include shopping, gardening, moving furniture, climbing stairs and lifting ourselves out of a chair or bath. If we participate in sporting activities, either recreational or competitive, we may require greater strength and endurance than we normally need to perform our daily tasks efficiently. In everyday life we never need to lift the heavy weights a power lifter needs to move; neither do we need the endurance to perform thousands of press-ups or sit-ups. Our primary aim should be that our muscles are strong enough to perform our daily tasks with a little in reserve.

Strong muscles will help us to maintain the correct alignment of our skeleton; weak muscles

**Figure 1.2 Curvatures of the spine**

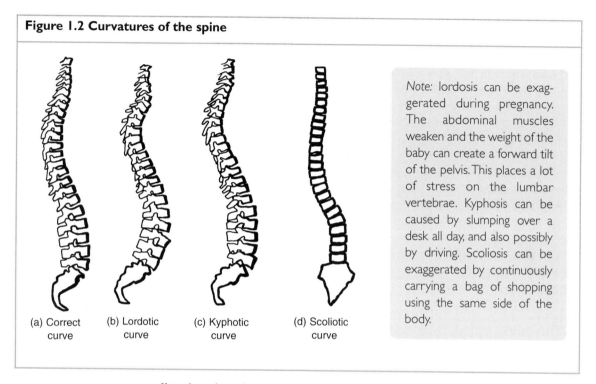

(a) Correct curve    (b) Lordotic curve    (c) Kyphotic curve    (d) Scoliotic curve

*Note:* lordosis can be exaggerated during pregnancy. The abdominal muscles weaken and the weight of the baby can create a forward tilt of the pelvis. This places a lot of stress on the lumbar vertebrae. Kyphosis can be caused by slumping over a desk all day, and also possibly by driving. Scoliosis can be exaggerated by continuously carrying a bag of shopping using the same side of the body.

may cause an uneven pull to be placed on our skeleton. Our muscles work in pairs, i.e. as one contracts and works, the opposite muscle relaxes. If one of the pair is contracted or worked too frequently and becomes too strong, and the other is not worked sufficiently or is allowed to become weaker, then our joints will be pulled out of correct alignment. This may cause injury or create postural defects such as rounded shoulders or excessive curvature of the spine. These defects are illustrated in figure 1.2. An imbalance of strength in the abdominal and opposing muscles of the back (the erector spinae) can cause an exaggerated curve or hollowing of the lumbar vertebrae (lordosis). An imbalance in the strength of the muscles of the chest (the pectorals) and the muscles between the shoulder blades (the rhomboids and trapezius) can cause rounded shoulders and a humping of the thoracic spine (kyphosis). An imbalance in the strength of the muscles on each side of the back can cause a sideways curvature of the thoracic spine (scoliosis). All our muscles should be kept sufficiently strong to maintain a correct posture. Our lifestyle, however, may demand that we specifically target certain muscles more than others to compensate for the imbalances caused by our work and daily activities. For the majority of individuals with a sedentary lifestyle, it is worthwhile strengthening the abdominal muscles, the muscles in between the shoulder blades (trapezius and rhomboids), and possibly the muscles of the back (erector spinae).

Training for muscular strength and endurance will also improve the tone of our muscles. Toned muscles are firmer and more shapely and provide us with an improved body shape and physical appearance. If our body is toned and taut we may have a more positive self-image, which, in turn, enhances our psychological well-being and self-confidence.

Finally, muscular strength and endurance training can also improve the strength and health of our bones and joints. The muscles have to contract and pull against the bones to create movement and lift the resistance. In response, our tendons, which attach the muscles to the bone across the joint, and our ligaments, which attach bone to bone across the joint, will become stronger. In the long term our joints will become stronger, more stable, and at less risk from injury. Increased calcium can be deposited and stored by the bones, preventing them from becoming brittle and reducing the risk of osteoporosis. Muscular strength and endurance training can therefore provide many long-lasting benefits which can extend the quality of our life for a number of years.

## Summary of the long-term benefits of muscular strength and endurance training

- Increased bone density (more calcium laid down).
- Decreased risk of osteoporosis.
- Improved performance of sporting and recreational activities.
- Efficient performance of daily tasks.
- Improved body shape ad tone.
- Improved self-image.
- Improved self-confidence.
- Stronger muscles, ligaments and tendons, which are more supportive to movement.

## How can we improve our muscular strength and endurance?

Strength training is traditionally achieved by performing exercises that require us to lift heavy and near maximal resistances for a short period of time (high resistance and low repetitions). Endurance exercises require a lighter resistance to be lifted, but for an extended period of time (low resistance and high repetitions).

The types of activities that promote strength and endurance require a more isolated focus on the specific muscles. Weight training is a typical training mode, although callisthenic exercises such as Press-ups, Sit-ups etc. that require us to lift our body weight can be equally effective. These activities need to be performed approximately two to three times a week for sufficient improvement to be made. The resistance lifted should promote a fatigued feeling in the muscle after anything between 7 and 25 repetitions. The gains achieved by an individual will be determined by the number of repetitions they are able to perform: the lower the number of reps an individual is able to perform the more the gains will be to muscular strength; the more repetitions an individual is able to perform the more the gains will be for muscular endurance. The recommended training requirements for improving muscular strength and muscular endurance are outlined in table 1.3.

## How can we improve our muscular strength and endurance in an ETM programme?

Exercises which aim to isolate the work of specific muscle groups are effective. For some muscles, using our body weight as a resistance will be effective to improve strength and/or endurance. For example, Press-ups and Squats require the body weight to be lifted against the force of gravity, and Sit-ups, with the hands at the side of the head, utilise the arms (levers) as an additional weight for the abdominals to lift. However, in many instances it will be necessary to use equipment, such as body bars, dumbbells and bands, to create sufficient resistance to improve muscular strength and endurance. Exercises such as Barbell Curls and Lateral Raises, which are illustrated in chapter 9, will

| Table 1.3 | The recommended training requirements for improving muscular strength and endurance |
|---|---|
| *Frequency*<br>How often should we perform these activities | Working the same muscles on two to three occasions per week should be sufficient. |
| *Intensity*<br>How hard should we be working? | To improve our strength we need to work with a resistance which allows a low number of repetitions (approximately 5–7) to be performed. To improve our endurance we need to work with a slightly lower resistance which allows us to perform a slightly higher number of repetitions (approximately 12–25). Working with a resistance which allows us to perform between 7 and 12 repetitions will initially provide some improvement in both strength and endurance.<br><br>**Note**: the exercises should be performed at a moderate rate and achieve failure (i.e. not being able to perform another repetition) in the prescribed repetition range. |
| *Time*<br>How long should we sustain these activities for? | This will depend on the level of fitness of participants, the number of muscle groups worked, and the aims of the individual. As an approximate guideline, between 10 and 40 minutes (excluding warm-up and warm-down) should be sufficient to achieve a whole body approach and train all the major muscle groups. |
| *Type*<br>What types of activities are most effective? | Lifting weights or working with other resistances such as bands or body weight are effective. Exercises to improve muscular strength and endurance are illustrated and explained in chapter 9. Aim for a balanced whole body approach using between 8 and 12 different exercises. |

not be effective unless external resistance is provided.

## How can we cater for different abilities?

Muscular strength and endurance exercises can be intensified progressively by increasing the length of the levers being moved, moving at a slower pace, and using an external resistance. Less fit participants should be encouraged to progress more steadily by using these methods singularly, i.e. they may need to perform Side Leg Raises with a straight leg, but at a moderate tempo and without external resistance.

Fitter participants can be encouraged to use all three of these progressive methods together, i.e. they could perform Side Leg Raises with a straight leg, at a slow pace and with an ankle weight attached. This would provide them with a greater challenge.

## What is motor fitness?

Motor fitness is a skill-related component of fitness and refers to a number of inter-related factors including agility, balance, speed, co-ordination, reaction time, and power.

## Why do we need motor fitness?

Motor fitness requires the effective transmission and management of messages and responses between the central nervous system (the brain and spinal cord) and the peripheral nervous system (sensory and motor). The peripheral nervous system collects information via the sensory system, the central nervous system receives and processes this information and sends an appropriate response via the motor system, which initiates the appropriate response.

Motor fitness is more applicable to the sportsperson, however it can have an indirect effect on the improvement of our fitness in the other health-related fitness components. Development of specific skills can improve our performance of certain activities. Skilful movements are more efficient: if we move skilfully we can improve the effectiveness of the activities we perform and by learning to perform exercises with the correct technique, we will reduce the risk of injury that can be caused by moving with our body in poor alignment. Therefore, improved motor fitness will maximise both the safety and effectiveness of our performance.

## How can we improve our motor fitness?

Managing our body weight, manoeuvring our centre of gravity, co-ordinating our body movements, moving at different speeds, in different directions and at different intensities, will all in the long term contribute to improving our motor fitness. If we want to improve our motor fitness, we must specifically and repeatedly train the aspect we wish to improve. If we want to perform a quick, co-ordinated sequence of movements, we need to perform the specific movements that make up that sequence and we may need to train ourselves to develop the necessary skills, which in this example are speed and co-ordination. In order to train ourselves, we should break down the sequence into smaller components and perform each component in isolation and at a slow pace. By progressively linking one component to another, and moving at a quicker pace, we will, in time, develop the necessary skills to perform the whole sequence at the appropriate speed. We will therefore have improved our motor fitness.

However, if we wish to learn to walk the tightrope, we need to develop different skills in a different way. Balance will be a very important skill to develop for this activity; performing our co-ordinated sequence of movements will not assist our balance on the tightrope. Training to improve our motor fitness must specifically relate to the activities we need or want to perform, but we must ensure that we are not put off if we cannot do something initially. In time, we can all learn the necessary skills to perform any activity. The key is to break down the skill and allow ourselves the time to develop it slowly. A good teacher will break down the skill for us and encourage us as we practise and develop.

## How can we improve our motor fitness in an ETM programme?

All ETM programmes will require the development of certain skills for the exercises to be carried out safely, and in time to the music: moving rhythmically can be challenging enough for some participants. Certain themed classes will require specific skills to be developed: a funk class may emphasise co-ordination; a sculpt class may emphasise power; a stretch class may emphasise balance. Therefore, the specific improvements required will be dependent to a great extent on the type of programme.

## Summary of the benefits of physical fitness

By performing the appropriate types of activities we can improve each component of physical fitness: our heart, lungs and circulatory system will become more efficient, allowing us to perform activities for a longer period of time, and without becoming excessively breathless; our muscles will become stronger giving us a more toned appearance and improving our posture; our joints will become more flexible

and allow us to move with greater ease, more efficiency and better control. By improving our physical fitness we are making endless contributions to enhancing our quality of life.

But, more importantly, by developing our physical fitness we are making a significant contribution to improving our overall health and total fitness. Being physically fit will keep our heart healthy and decrease the risk of coronary heart disease; it will keep our bones and joints healthy, preventing the onset of osteoporosis, and allowing us to maintain a full range of motion; it will keep our muscles strong, providing greater support to our skeleton; and it will also help us to manage our body weight. Ultimately, we should live a longer and fuller life!

## What is total fitness?

Overall health, or total fitness, requires us to be socially, mentally, emotionally, nutritionally, and medically fit, as well as being physically fit. Our level of physical fitness will affect our overall health or total fitness, however total fitness requires a little bit more than just taking part in regular physical activity: it demands that we also pay attention to our lifestyle, our diet, our stress levels, our emotions, our ability to communicate, and recognise that sometimes it is important for us to simply relax and recuperate. ETM is an effective way of improving the components of total fitness.

## What is social fitness?

Social fitness involves interaction and communication with people. If we improve our physical fitness then we are making ourselves physically more able to participate in a greater range of social activities (sporting and recreational) and can, therefore, potentially improve our social fitness.

## How can ETM improve our social fitness?

ETM appears to be particularly effective for improving our social fitness. This may be due to the fact that it is a group activity, which naturally encourages networking and friendships to blossom among class members. Indeed, the social activities which occur after the session are all due to relationships being developed. Some classes use partner work, themed routines and group activities specifically to lighten the atmosphere and encourage interaction among class members. Either way, it is evident that ETM enhances communication and promotes the development of friendships between a wide range of participants.

## What is mental and emotional fitness?

Mental and emotional fitness refers to our psychological well-being. The pressures of daily life can have a negative effect on our mental and emotional fitness causing us to feel tired, anxious and stressed. When we feel stressed we stimulate the release of hormones that prepare us for fight or flight. As a consequence we release sugars into the blood stream to provide energy for the necessary physical action. However, all too often we do not take action (fight or flight) and instead stew on our problems. This has a negative effect on our health because sugars are released which can potentially contribute to atherosclerosis (furring up of the artery walls). Stress is therefore a contributory factor to a number of minor and major diseases, including high blood pressure, coronary heart disease, irritable bowel syndrome and anxiety, so it is wise to take some precautionary measures to reduce our stress levels.

## How can ETM improve our mental and emotional fitness?

There are a number of reasons why regular ETM can help with stress management. First, the physical exertion necessary to perform exercises provides us with an excellent way of releasing pressure and tension. Second, when we are exercising and when we are listening to music our minds will be distracted from any daily hassles or worries. Third, when we take part in aerobic exercise, we increase the circulation of endorphins, a hormone which gives us an enhanced feeling of well-being. This feeling can last for much longer than the duration of the actual exercise session. Finally, the long-term improvements to our body shape and physical appearance can enhance self-esteem, self-image and self-confidence. If we feel confident about ourselves we will act confidently, which can have a tremendous effect on our psychological well-being.

Most ETM classes include a specific cool-down component, and within that component stretching exercises are used that can have a relaxing effect on the mind and body. In addition, specific relaxation techniques can be used to create a relaxed atmosphere; themed music can have a soothing effect on the mind; and specific stretch and relax classes that focus on the mind and body are also becoming more popular. These are particularly effective for improving emotional and mental fitness and appropriate activities for this type of session are discussed in later chapters.

## What is nutritional fitness?

Nutritional fitness requires us to eat a balanced diet. The foods we eat will affect how much energy we have and will also affect our health and well-being. It is worth remembering that there are no bad foods, just poor diets. It is essential that we eat a balanced diet from the main food groups: carbohydrates (pasta, potatoes, bread); fats (cheese, milk, butter); proteins (beans, pulses, meat); vitamins and minerals (vegetables and fruit); and water. We should also ensure that the quantity of food we consume is appropriate to meet our requirements.

## How can ETM improve our nutritional fitness?

Taking part in regular physical activity can make us more aware of the food we eat and more conscious of our diet. There are many textbooks devoted to the subject of total fitness and some of these are listed at the end of this book. The following are some general rules only for improving our diet.

- Eat less saturated fat: too much will increase risk of high cholesterol and increase furring of the artery walls.
- Eat less sugar: too much will cause tooth decay and promote the risk of adult onset diabetes.
- Eat less salt: too much will potentially elevate blood pressure.
- Eat more complex carbohydrates: too little will lower our energy levels.
- Eat sufficient fibre: too little will potentially cause constipation and other bowel disorders.
- Eat a sufficient calorie intake: too little will slow down our metabolism and make us feel lethargic; too much will make us put on weight and will be stored as body fat.
- Drink more water: too little fluid will cause dehydration, potential heat stroke and place unnecessary stress on the heart.

After exercise the appetite is increased due to the energy and calories expended during the workout. The best time to replenish our glycogen stores (stored carbohydrate that we need for energy) is within two hours of activity. However, because many of us use exercise to assist with our weight management, it is worthwhile preparing a healthy and nutritional snack to eat after our activity. This will possibly reduce the temptation for us to purchase and consume a less nutritional snack. If we can plan our exercise programme, we can also plan our diet.

## What is medical fitness?

Medical fitness is our state of health and well-being. It requires our body to be in optimal working order, that is, not injured or ill. Improvements in all the components of physical fitness contribute significantly to this aspect of our total fitness.

## How can ETM improve our medical fitness?

Regular activity and keeping physically fit can reduce the risk of many medical problems, including: high blood pressure, coronary heart disease, osteoporosis, obesity, stress-related illnesses, and many others. In addition, regular exercise and our improved fitness can encourage us to eat healthier, manage stress more effectively and maintain a healthy body composition. Attending an ETM class may also provide a substitute for other less beneficial social activities. This, in turn, may help us to cut down or remove habits that have an adverse effect on our health, such as smoking, drinking excessive alcohol, or eating too much of the less nutritious foods.

A well-structured and effective ETM programme has the potential to bring about significant improvements in physical and total fitness. Later chapters in this book discuss how to structure the session to maximise these improvements for all participants.

## Summary of the benefits of ETM

ETM will potentially:

- improve all components of physical fitness
- assist with weight management
- promote social interaction
- encourage a healthier lifestyle
- assist with stress management
- improve self-esteem and confidence with physical appearance
- enhance feelings of well-being
- improve overall health.

# MUSIC AND CHOREOGRAPHY

## Why use music?

Most people enjoy listening to music, and many enjoy actually exercising to music (performing a routine of exercises to a piece of music) or exercising with music (having music playing in the background while exercising). Exercising to music can be fun and very motivating and can enhance both the atmosphere created and the performance of participants. Some of the possible advantages and disadvantages of using music are listed in table 2.1.

## What type of music is appropriate?

Selecting the right type of music is very time-consuming and challenging. The ETM teacher needs to be aware of the variety of music that is available and sensitive to the preferences of the participants for different types of music. They should consider the age and ability of the participants, the type of class and the component of the class they are choosing music for. All of these factors affect the type of music which is selected.

| Table 2.1 | The advantages and disadvantages of using music |
|---|---|
| **Advantages of using music** | **Disadvantages of using music** |
| *Creates atmosphere* <br> Lively and fun music will create an inspirational atmosphere for the more active (aerobic) components of the session; a strong beat will dictate a good pace for muscular strength and endurance training; slow and melodious music will create a calm and soothing atmosphere for the more relaxing components. | *Creates the wrong atmosphere* <br> If music is too slow and laborious it will not inspire participants to move actively in the aerobic components; a weak beat used for muscular strength and endurance components will not dictate a good working pace; a strong beat in the stretch components may create bouncing and distract from the desired relaxed atmosphere. |
| *Motivating* <br> It can create a rhythm to work to and inspire participants to keep working. If different types of music are used all ages can be catered for and will enjoy the session. | *Can demotivate or overmotivate* <br> If participants do not like the music chosen they may find the session boring and uninspiring. Alternatively, motivating music played when participants are tired may encourage them to work hard when they should slow down. |
| *Dictates the pace of the session* <br> Well-paced music will allow all participants to perform exercises at a safe and effective pace, assisting with control of the session. | *Dictates an inappropriate pace* <br> If music is too fast participants may not be able to keep up; if it is too slow movements will be lethargic. The speed of music one selects should take account of the participants' different body types and abilities, all of which affect their ability to work to a prescribed beat. |

| **Table 2.1** | **The advantages and disadvantages of using music cont.** |
|---|---|
| *Assists planning of the session* <br> Knowing the duration of a specific music tape allows the teacher to plan the sessions and each component safely and effectively to meet the needs of the participants. | *Can make the session too rigid* <br> The teacher must always be prepared to adapt the session if the group is unable to cope. They should also be prepared to adapt specific exercises to accommodate the variety of individuals within the session. |
| *Enjoyment* <br> Hearing a piece of music that you like listening to is inspirational and fun and may encourage commitment to an exercise programme. | *Monotonous* <br> If variety of music is insufficient to accommodate for different tastes, or if music tapes are not changed regularly, commitment may lessen. |
| *A cost-effective investment* <br> Most people enjoy exercising to music and are attracted to sessions where music is played. | *Expensive* <br> Music licences (PPL and PRS), music tapes and audio equipment are all expensive. The teacher must purchase a sufficient variety of music tapes for variety in the session. It is usually more cost-effective for teachers with a large number of classes to subscribe to one of the music agencies (Pure Energy or Telstar). |
| *Assists coaching of the session* <br> Moving in time to the music and knowing the sequence of moves will help maintain control of participants' movements, and can assist the teacher with cueing and instructions and provide them with more time and opportunities to move around to observe and correct individuals. | *Can distract from coaching* <br> If music is too loud participants may be unable to hear instructions and coaching points; if music is too quiet it may reduce enjoyment and participants may be unable to follow. Additionally, if the teacher gets carried away by a piece of music they may become too concerned with their own performance and forget to observe and correct participants. |

There is a variety of different types of music which can be used for ETM. House, Garage, Funk, R&B, hiphop, rock, pop, Hollywood themes, and lots more have all been used by teachers to create different themes for their ETM sessions and masterclasses. The most popular and traditional rhythm used in ETM sessions is 4/4 time. This is suitable for most activities and is easiest for most people to move to. There are, however, a number of different rhythms (e.g. 3/4 and 6/8 time) which can be used if the teacher and participants are sufficiently skilled to hear and work to the changes in the music phrase.

## Music for warming up

The music used at the start of the session will establish the atmosphere and mental attitude throughout the class. It is wise to use an uplifting piece of music to establish the appropriate atmosphere, however care must be taken to ensure that the music speed allows for full control of all movements during this preparatory component of the class, otherwise injury may occur. It may be useful to perform the initial mobility and pulse-raising exercises at half time and/or through a small range of motion to ensure that sufficient control is maintained. As the body gets warmer, the exercises can be performed at a faster tempo and through a greater range of motion without placing the body at risk.

Newcomers to ETM will generally need to work at a slower pace than experienced exercisers; they need longer to warm up and more time to execute movements correctly. Fitter participants can generally warm up to a faster piece of music because their bodies respond more effectively to warming up activities and they are able to control their movements more effectively.

## Music for cardio-vascular training

The music used for this component needs to be vigorous with a strong beat. The music must motivate participants sufficiently to keep working and create a fun atmosphere. The music used should also allow for a sufficient variety of movements to be used in a sequence; too many high-impact jogging movements or too many deep squatting movements performed in succession may be too stressful for the joints. It is advisable to plan a mixture of high- and low-impact movements and to combine these with travelling movements to create sufficient variations of joint stresses. The music selected should allow for this variety of movement.

Newcomers to ETM may initially need to work at a slightly slower, more moderate pace to ensure they move through a safe range of motion and with sufficient control of movements. As their fitness increases they will be able to perform the movements through a greater range of motion and with greater control, and faster music can progressively be introduced. At all times care must be taken to ensure that the speed of music is not so fast that adequate control of movements is lost by participants. The teacher should also be aware of all participants and ensure that they are not

being carried along with the atmosphere and overworking. Leaving the class feeling exhausted may deter them from attending another ETM session.

Fitter participants can move quite easily and execute movements at a slightly faster pace. However, if the music used is too fast and up tempo even they may struggle to achieve a full range of motion. Ultimately, the music selected for this component should always promote safe and effective movement from participants. It should also reflect the theme of the class.

## Music for muscular strength and endurance training

A strong, regular and not too vigorous beat of music is ideal for this component. This will help to maintain the speed at which exercises are performed and can help keep participants moving at the same time. The music used for this component should also allow for work to different beats (slow and quick). It is useful if the teacher is able to vary the tempo (i.e. lift for two counts and lower for two counts or lift for three counts and lower for one count to alter the effect of the exercise). Working at a slower pace may reduce the amount of repetitions that participants are able to perform and may therefore bring about different training benefits.

Newcomers to ETM may initially need to work at a slightly slower pace to allow adequate time for them to perform the exercises through the full range of motion and with sufficient control. As their skill and fitness level increases, they should be able to work at a slightly faster pace while still working through the full range of motion.

Fitter participants are generally able to work at a slightly faster pace. However, often it is the slower movements which are more demanding, since the muscles have to contract and work for longer. It is advisable to provide a greater number of speed variations for a fitter group and ultimately the pace of the music can be slightly more up tempo.

## Music for stretching

The pace of music used for the stretching components of the class needs to be fairly slow to ensure that stretch positions are not bounced or pulsed, which could create overstretching and cause damage to the muscles. For the warm-up/preparatory stretch, the music cannot be too slow: if the music used is too slow, the atmosphere created and motivation to continue working may be lost. It is wise for teachers to use a piece of music which maintains motivation, and to ensure that they instruct participants carefully, so that stretch positions are not reached too quickly or bounced.

The music used for stretching at the end of the class should be slower and more relaxing. It should allow for stretch positions to be held still and for the mind and body to be given time to relax and unwind. It is wise to choose a piece of music that has few vocals and no strong beat. Instrumental and classical themes are recommended for creating the appropriate atmosphere.

## Should the teacher select the music before they plan the exercises?

It is generally recommended that less experienced teachers plan the exercises for each component of the class before they select the music. This will ensure that the pace of music is suitable to perform the planned exercises. It will also ensure that the desired aims for each component of the session are achieved.

More experienced teachers will be able to adapt the exercises (intensity, rate and range of motion) to fit the music and still achieve the desired safe and effective aims. All teachers are advised to read the chapters that relate to the structure and planning of specific components of the class to assist with the selection of music.

## What is an appropriate music speed?

All music has a regular beat which dictates the speed at which the exercises should be performed. Teachers of ETM should select music very carefully since participants will vary in their height, weight, body type, body composition, fitness and skill level. Each of these factors will affect whether the person is able to perform a specific exercise to the beat of music prescribed.

Lean participants and participants with an adequate skill and fitness level will generally be able to move at a fairly fast tempo; less fit participants, specialist groups, curvaceous body types, and participants with less motor skills will need to work at a slower pace. The easiest way for a teacher to accommodate this is to select a moderately-paced piece of music, i.e. in the middle of the recommended speed ranges for each component, which are outlined in table 2.2 (*see* page 21). They should also offer a variety of alternatives to alter the range of motion and intensity for each exercise to allow for safe and effective performance.

In addition, some exercises take longer to perform than others. Exercises which require a large range of motion to be performed, for example a Squat or Lunge, will take longer to perform through the full range of motion and will therefore need a slower music beat. Alternatively, exercises which work through a small range of motion, for example jogging and marching, can be performed at a faster beat. If a combination of large and small range of motion exercises are used in the same sequence, the teacher should plan the exercises so that the necessary variations of speed are allowed, for example using the quick beat for smaller movements and the slow beat for larger movements. This will ensure that the exercises are executed effectively and through the full range of motion; it will also maintain work to the appropriate beat of the music. Once again, selecting a moderately-paced piece of music will make it easier for the teacher to plan and adapt. It should be noted that the speed ranges suggested are only guidelines: some people may need to work slower and some may be

| Table 2.2 | Guidelines for selecting music of an appropriate speed |
|---|---|
| **Component of the session** | **Approximate guidelines for the speed of music** |
| *Warm-up*<br>The music used for mobility and pulse raising should build progressively. Ideally, the music used for preparatory stretching should be slightly slower. | 120–134 bpm |
| *Cardio-vascular (aerobic) training*<br>The music used at the start and at the end of the cardio-vascular training component should be of a slightly slower pace to allow for an adequate build-up and cool-down of intensity. (Newcomers, tall people and people with large body frames are less likely to achieve a fuller range of motion, so if the music is too fast a more moderate pace, which allows a mix of impact, will provide a safer workout.) | Low impact 125–140 bpm<br>High impact 135–150 bpm<br><br>*Safety note*: it is advisable to use a moderate pace of music that allows for a mix of high and low impact. |
| *Muscular strength and endurance (toning and resistance) training*<br>If weights are used the music will need to be slightly slower to allow for the equipment to be moved safely and effectively. | 110–125 bpm |
| *Step training*<br>The speed of music will also be dependent on the height of the step and the height, body frame and experience of participants. | 120–125 bpm |
| *Post-workout stretching, relaxation*<br>Music without vocals can be more relaxing at the end of the session and for use in a mind and body session. | 80–110 bpm |
| *Re-mobilise*<br>Care should be taken not to end the session in a manic fashion; a gentle enlivener is all that is needed. | 120–125 bpm |

able to perform faster. It is a good idea for a coach to seek constant feedback from the participants to check whether they are able to move at the speed being dictated.

## How can music be used?

There are a number of ways that music can be used throughout an ETM session. Ideally, all movements should be planned to the music to maximise the effects of using music. However, in the slower more relaxing components it is acceptable to have music as background to create the atmosphere without dictating the pace.

### Background

This is where music is played but the movements are not executed in time to the music, nor are any changes in movement cued to the music phrase. This approach is traditionally adopted during the post-workout stretch and relaxation components of the session. It can also be used when circuit training to music, however it is often more appropriate if changes in the music phrase are used to manage movement from one station to another and to cue the next exercise.

### Beat and phrasing

This is where any changes of a movement sequence are planned to occur at the start of a music phrase and the movements are also performed to the beat of the music. This approach should be adopted through most components of the session if it is to be called ETM: using music just as background is exercising *with* music, not to music.

To identify where changes in the music phrase occur, listen to a piece of popular music (which is normally 4/4 time). Generally speaking, eight beats will make up one music phrase. The first beat of each phrase is usually stronger than the other beats and almost marks the start of a new sentence in the music. Once you are satisfied that you can hear the changes of the music phrase, write down each set of eight counts that occur throughout the whole track. This will take a bit of practice if you are unfamiliar with breaking down music. Table 2.3 provides guidelines on how a sequence of moves can be planned to fit with musical phrases. ETM teacher training courses also include practice in how to do this.

| Table 2.3 | Planning exercises to fit with musical phrases | |
|---|---|---|
| *Music counts* | *Exercise* | *Teaching points* |
| 2 sets of 8 counts (16) | March on the spot. | Land lightly, not stamping the feet. |
| 2 sets of 8 counts (16) | Step and tap and roll the shoulders back to mobilise the shoulders. | Keep the body lifted and the knees unlocked. Control movements of the shoulder. Progressively move through a larger range of motion. |
| 2 sets of 8 counts (16) | Squat/plié in place. | Knees in line with toes and not locking the knees. |
| 2 sets of 8 counts (16) | Side bend to mobilise the spine. | Lean directly to the side, not bending too far over. |

## Verse and chorus choreography

This is where the music is broken down and the introduction, verses, chorus and any instrumentals are identified. A sequence of movements are planned to be performed and repeated for the verse and another sequence of movements are planned to be repeated for the chorus. All changes of movement should occur to the phrase of the music.

This approach can be ideal when working with those less skilled at exercising to music. If the exercises selected are simple, and changes to movements less frequent, they can work effectively and stay working to the music phrase. It also provides more repetition enabling them to learn and memorise a sequence of moves. If they are familiar with the movements they are about to perform they are generally able to concentrate more on their technique and posture. This will enhance the safety and effectiveness of their performance.

This approach is most easily used in the cardio-vascular component, however it can also work effectively in the warm-up, cool-down and muscular strength and endurance components. Table 2.4 provides guidelines on how to plan a sequence of moves to the verse and chorus.

## Adding on choreography

In its most simplistic form, add-on choreography is about adding one move to another move. For example, one move is performed for a set number of counts or until it has been mastered by the group and then another move is added and so on. Once a complete sequence of moves has been performed, they can be broken down and performed for fewer repetitions (see pyramid technique) so that a sequence of moves are performed for a specific count of music. The technique can be repeated with a new set of moves. The second sequence can be broken down using a pyramid to form a second sequence. Once two sequences have been mastered, then can be added together. See table

| Table 2.4 | Planning exercises to the verse and chrous | |
|---|---|---|
| *Music counts* | *Exercise* | *Teaching points* |
| Intro: 2 sets of 8 counts (16) | March in place. | Land lightly, not stamping the feet. |
| Verse: 2 sets of 8 counts (16) | Grapevine right and left. | Lead with the heel, knees in line with the toes, chest lifted. |
| Chorus: 2 sets of 8 counts (16) | Walk forwards for four counts and backwards for four counts. | Heel toe action, not locking the knees. |
| Instrumental: 2 sets of 8 counts (16) | March in place and half turn to face the back wall. | As above – marching. |
| Verse: 2 sets of 8 counts (16) | Repeat Grapevines. | As above – Grapevines. |
| Chorus: 2 sets of 8 counts (16) | Repeat walks forwards and backwards. | As above – walks. |

2.5 and the sample choreography plans at the end of this chapter.

The number of sequences which can be broken down and added together will depend on the skills of the group and the complexity of the sequence patterns selected. This approach to choreography is traditionally used in the cardio-vascular training component. It can also work effectively in the warm-up. Table 2.5 provides guidelines on how to add on a sequence of moves.

# How can choreography be broken down?

## Visual preview and holding pattern

A holding pattern is a movement that the class can perform while the teacher demonstrates the next development of that move.

For example:

**Holding pattern:** Class perform leg curls facing the front (8 count)

**Visual preview:** Teacher demonstrates leg curls with turns to face the right, back, left and

| Table 2.5 | Planning an add on choreography sequence | |
|---|---|---|
| *Music counts* | *Exercise* | *Teaching points* |
| 2 sets of 8 counts (16) | Grapevine right and left (8 counts) Mambo right (4 counts) and jump to the right (4 counts). | Lead with heel. Do not lock the knee. Heels down on the jump. |
| 2 sets of 8 counts (16) | Perform whole sequence moving to left first (16 counts). | As above. |
| Total of 32 counts | The complete sequence works to an even 32-count phrase. *How to break down and add on:* 1 Teach and perform grapevines. 2 Perform Grapevine right and left and then march for 8 counts. Perform Grapevine left and then right and march for 8 counts. 3 As above but instead of marching for the last set of 4 counts jump in place. 4 As above but instead of marching for the first set of 4 counts perform mambo. 5 As above but travel the jump in the the direction of the initial **Grapevine**. *Note*: the speed at which each of these move-ments can be added together will be dependent on the ability of the group. It may be necessary to repeat each stage a number of times before preceding to the next stage. | |

front of the room so that a full circle of leg curls are performed (8 count).

## Pyramid

A pyramid is where the number of repetitions of an exercise or sequence of exercises are reduced sequentially to make up the final sequence.
For example:
$1 \times 32$ grapevine right and left
$1 \times 32$ box step right lead
Repeat left

## Reverse pyramid

Reduce pyramid to $1 \times 16$ counts all above
Reduce pyramid to $1 \times 8$ counts all above.
Reverse pyramiding is a variation of the above. Instead of decreasing, increase the repetition. Using a step, perform a diagonally travelling up tap step – 1 right, 1 left. For example: (8 counts). Increase reps to 2 tap ups right and left (16 counts).

# How can choreography be varied?

Quite often, teachers will avidly seek new movements to include in their class. Constantly searching for new movements is often time-consuming and not always successful. It is worth noting that in reality there are only a certain number of directions our joints can move in, which will affect the movements we are able to perform. However, this need not limit our choreography patterns: it is often more effective to find ways of varying the movements we already use. This can be achieved by the following types of variations.

- Combining the different movements together to form a new sequence for one music phrase.
- Varying the speed of some of the movements in a sequence, i.e. run, run, hold and repeat. This uses the quick, quick, slow rhythm.

- Moving the sequence in a different direction: forwards, backwards, sideways, to a diagonal, in a circle, or in a figure of eight, depending on the movement being used.
- Varying the arm lines used.
- Using a turn to vary the body part leading the move, e.g. galloping right for two counts, pivot half turn and galloping left for two counts and march for four counts. Repeat to return to face front.
- Performing an exercise or part of a sequence of exercises in a different exercise mode, e.g. low impact, high impact, power move etc.

A whole range of basic exercises are illustrated in later chapters of this book. Ideas for varying and progressing each exercise are also explained. Teachers will find their own way of varying these movements and creating their own choreography with experience and practice.

## Basic – 16 count choreography sequences

- Walk forward $\times 4$ and 2 calf raises
- Repeat back = 16 counts.

- Walk forward $\times 4$ and 2 jumping jacks
- Repeat back = 16 counts

- Walk forward $\times 4$ and 2 side lunges
- Repeat back = 16 counts

- Walk forward $\times 4$ and 2 pony steps
- Repeat back = 16 counts

Walks can be varied by walking to the side.
- Scoop forward $\times 4$ and back $\times 4 = 16$ counts.

Scoops can be varied and travelled to the diagonal.
- Grapevine right and left, 1 box step forward, 1 box step backwards.
- Repeat left = 16 counts

- Grapevine right and left, mambo $\times 2$
- Repeat left = 16 counts

| Table 2.6 | Lesson Plan: Aerobic/Cardio vascular (Mixed ability) – simple chroreography | | |
|---|---|---|---|
| Music counts | Exercise Description | Choreography Progression 1 | Choreography Progression 2 |
| 1 × 32 | **Sequence A** <br> Grapevine 1 × right <br> Grapevine 1 × left <br> Box step 2 × forward <br><br> Repeat left lead | Add jump <br><br> 1 box forward and 1 box backwards | Add jump <br><br> 2 back box step turning (still travel to front on 1st box step but facing back of class front |
| 1 × 32 <br> 1 × 32 | **Choreography Break down:** <br> Grapevine R <br> Box step R <br> Repeat left <br><br> **Pyramid** down all above <br> 1 × 16 R and L <br> 1 × 8 R and L | | |
| 1 × 32 | **Sequence B** <br> Walk forward × 4 right lead <br> Calf raise × 2 <br> Lunge backs × 4 <br><br> Repeat walking backwards | Jog forward <br> Bounce calf raise <br> Single, single, double lunge | Same <br> Same <br> Single, single <br> Lunge kick ball change |
| 1 × 32 <br> 1 × 32 <br> 1 × 32 <br> 1 × 32 | **Breakdown:** <br> Walk forward and calf raise <br> Walk back and calf raise <br> Lunge back <br> Lunge back <br> (single, single, double) <br><br> **Add together** <br> To form B sequence <br><br> **Visual preview** <br> Lunge kick ball change to replace single, single, double. | | |
| | **Add-on sequence A and B together.** | | |
| 1 × 32 | Walk right (4 counts) <br> March (12 counts) <br><br> Repeat walking left | Gallop right <br> March (4 counts) <br> Mambo (4 count) | Same <br> Same <br> Mambo turn |
| 1 × 32 | Scoop forward × 4 <br> Scoop back × 4 <br> _ or full jump jacks × 8 <br> Repeat same | Scoop jump <br><br> Turn jacks to face back <br> Repeat to back | Scoop chasse |

- Grapevine right, turn step left. 4 × pony step
- Repeat left = 16 counts

Grapevine can be travelled to diagonals
- Gallop right and jump in place × 4
- Repeat left = 16 counts

- Gallop right and jump in small circle
- Repeat left = 16 counts

- Gallop right and 2 × mambos
- Repeat left = 16 counts

**Summary of basic moves and choreography tools:**
There are only a few basic moves that most choreography develops from. These include:
1. March
2. Side step
3. Heel dig
4. Calf raise
5. Back lunge

6. Squat
7. Leg curl

To add variation to choreography teachers can use the following choreography tools.
1. Level length
2. Range of motion (R.O.M.)
3. Reps
4. Rhythm
5. Travel
6. Turns
7. Arm line
8. Direction
9. Impact
10. Combine with a new move
11. Change lead legs

Table 2.7 provides an example of some basic guideline for adding variation to choreography using some of these tools for three of the basic moves.

| Table 2.7 | Developing basic choreography | | |
|---|---|---|---|
| Choreography tools | Step touch | Heel dig | Back lunge |
| Lever length | Hamstring curl | Knee lift or straight leg raise | N/A |
| Reps | Double side step | Double knee lift | Double back lunge |
| R.O.M. | Grapevine | Double knee crossing over in front | Back kicks |
| Rhythm | Syncopate double side step to chasse | Heel dig – quick, quick, slow | Single, single double |
| Impact | Add Jump to any of above | Add jump | Spotty dogs |
| Travel | Forwards or back | Travel forward or back Travel 4 heel toe to right then left | Back kicks travelling back |
| Turn | 4 turning leg curls galloping turn gallop | _ turn on each knee lift to turn and travel | Turn back kicks in full circle |

# DESIGNING AN EXERCISE TO MUSIC PROGRAMME

PART **TWO**

# SAFETY IN THE EXERCISE ENVIRONMENT

## Who can attend an ETM session?

Everyone can benefit from attending an ETM session. Most people can quite easily be accommodated within a session, provided alternatives are offered to meet special requirements. However, some ETM sessions are quite high in intensity and do not cater specifically for persons with special requirements. Antenatal and postnatal women and older adults are two specific groups that are best advised to join a more specialist ETM class. In addition, some participants will need to obtain permission from their doctor before embarking on any programme of physical activity. This is to ensure that the exercise programme will be appropriate to meet their needs and that they will not be placing their well-being at risk by participating. They too are best advised to attend a more specialist, or lower level, class once permission is granted. Teachers should advise participants who answer yes to any of the health screening checks outlined in table 3.1 to check with their doctor prior to taking part in any physical activity.

## How can the teacher obtain this information from their target group?

There are three methods of gaining information from and about the target group.

- Visual (observing gender, age, body shape and size).
- Verbal (things you need to ask and be told by the participant).
- Written (questions).

| Table 3.1 | Health screening checks |
|---|---|

It is advisable to check with a doctor and seek their consent prior to commencing any physical activity if you:

- have high blood pressure, heart disease or cardio-vascular or respiratory problems
- have suffered from chest pains, especially if they are associated with light activity requiring minimal effort
- are prone to headaches, fainting or dizziness
- are pregnant, or have recently been pregnant
- have, or are recovering from, a joint problem or injury that may be aggravated by physical activity
- are taking medication or have any other medical condition
- have been recently ill
- are unused to exercise and over 35 years of age.

A few of the advantages and disadvantages of the different screening methods are identified in table 3.2.

Identifying the fitness goals and current health of individuals is only the first step in designing an appropriate ETM programme. It is also necessary to take into account the working environment, the equipment being used in the session, and the clothing being worn by participants. It is unsafe and ineffective to design a programme without identifying the peculiarities of different working environments, or to design a programme using equipment without understanding how the equipment should be lifted and manoeuvred.

| Table 3.2 | The advantages and disadvantages of different methods of screening | |
|---|---|---|
| *Method of screening* | *Advantages* | *Disadvantages* |
| Visual | • Quick.<br>• Can identify more personal issues without having to ask questions which may be embarrassing. | • Cannot identify all medical ailments visually. |
| Verbal | • Response is immediate.<br>• Information is up to date.<br>• Personal contact.<br>• Can probe and seek further information if necessary.<br>• Can highlight the importance of receiving the information.<br>• Can clarify and respond to any questions asked. | • Participants may be unwilling to provide personal information.<br>• Responses may not be completely true.<br>• There is no written record or proof of what has been asked, nor the response provided.<br>• Information provided may be forgotten.<br>• Time-consuming, since only one person can be spoken to at a time.<br>• Confidentiality – information should be obtained in private. |
| Written | • Permanent record of questions asked and responses provided.<br>• If the questionnaire used provides a yes or no response, concerns can be identified relatively quickly.<br>• Can screen more than one person at a time. | • Circumstances change, therefore written screening should be updated regularly.<br>• Screening forms need to be stored in a secure place and remain confidential.<br>• Questionnaires need to be worded carefully to obtain the accurate response.<br>• Information requested needs to encourage a concise response (yes/no). Wordy responses may be difficult to interpret and will take longer to read.<br>• Reading the responses to questionnaires is time-consuming. |

# What are the main environmental considerations?

## Floor surface

The floor surface is perhaps the most important consideration for the teacher of an ETM session. Ideally, the floor should be sprung so that impact forces from high-impact exercises are minimised. Performing high-impact exercises on a solid floor (concrete, or concrete with carpet) are contraindicated because the movements will not be cushioned and this may cause jarring and injury to the joints and shin splints.

If the floor surface is not sprung, the cardio-vascular exercises selected should be predominantly low impact to avoid placing the joints under too much stress. Alternatively, the session could be designed to feature more muscular strength and endurance work rather than cardio-vascular work. It is better to adapt the session than limit the opportunities for people to improve their fitness.

It is also essential to make sure that the floor surface is cleaned regularly, however it should not be so highly polished that the surface becomes slippery.

## Space

The size and shape of the room will affect the number of participants who can take part, the amount of travelling moves that can be used and the positioning of the teacher. Ideally, participants should be able to stand in one place, outstretch their arms in all directions and not come into contact with other people. If participants are able to reach another person, the room is probably overcrowded, which will make it difficult, and potentially unsafe, to use travelling movements. It will also make it difficult for the teacher to move around and correct participants. It is always advisable to limit class numbers and provide additional

sessions so that all participants can exercise safely and can be observed by the teacher.

The ideal environment is a wide rectangular room which allows for plenty of forwards and sideways travelling moves and plenty of space for the teacher to move around and correct. Long narrow rooms will limit forward travelling moves, and possibly sideways travelling moves if there are a lot of people in the room. The teacher will also need to vary their position frequently to see all participants in a long room; adopting one position throughout the session will limit their observation and prevent them from making essential corrections.

Teaching in a long narrow room will also limit the number of teaching fronts the teacher is able to use. The teacher should instruct primarily from the broadest sides of the room; using the narrow parts of the room will limit participants' observation and may prevent them from exercising safely and effectively. In this instance, the teacher will need to use their voice maximally to lead a movement and maintain effective control of the class.

## Mirrors

Mirrored walls are useful in many ways: they allow participants to observe their own performance and provide the opportunity for them to correct their own technique if they have sufficient knowledge of correct exercise alignment; they also provide a useful resource for the teacher, who can instruct a complex sequence of moves with their back to the group and still maintain some observation.

The biggest disadvantage of using mirrors is overuse. Facing the mirror for too long, and/or performing too many movements with their back to the group, prevents the teacher from moving around to other teaching positions and limits their observation of the participants. It also reduces direct eye contact and can potentially limit the rapport created between the teacher and the class.

Ideally, facing the mirror should be used in conjunction with other teaching positions where the teacher can move around to different points of the room and provide individual correction, motivation and praise, all of which can build class rapport and increase participants' confidence.

### Temperature

The temperature of the room will affect the structure and design of the main session. It will be unsafe and ineffective to perform a stretch class in a cold room; it will also be unsafe and ineffective to perform a very high-intensity cardio-vascular workout in an excessively hot room. The type of session provided will need to be adapted in these situations and general guidelines are outlined in table 3.3.

## What safety factors need to be considered when using equipment in an ETM session?

There is a variety of equipment that can be used in an ETM session: steps, slides, barbells, core balls, dumbbells, mats, bands, skipping ropes are just a few. Equipment will add variety to the session and can create a new approach to ETM. Some of these approaches are discussed in section three of this book.

When using equipment in an ETM session, the teacher should familiarise themselves with the manufacturers' guidelines to ensure that they use the equipment safely and effectively throughout the session. It may also be necessary for them to undertake further training to ensure they are qualified to use the equipment safely.

### Stacking, storage and maintenance of equipment

All equipment should be stored and stacked safely. Again the manufacturers' guidelines should be referred to. The following are recommended as general safety considerations.

- Store all barbells, dumbbells, ropes, bands in a large chest or in individual containers in the corner of the room.
- Ensure steps are not stacked too high; ideally have them caged to prevent them from falling and sliding across the room when the room is being used for other activities.
- Ensure that wires from electrical equipment are not trailing across the floor and that all plug fittings are secure.
- Stack exercise mats neatly at the side or back of the room. Ensure they are cleaned regularly and replaced when necessary.
- Regularly check the condition of weights and bands to ensure that all fixtures and fittings are secure.
- When equipment is in use ensure that it is spaced out safely (i.e. in a circuit or a step class do not position equipment too close together).
- Ensure that step risers are securely in place.
- Ensure that all equipment is lifted correctly.

### Lifting equipment

When moving equipment in an ETM session the teacher should ensure that all participants use the correct lifting technique – the Dead Lift. This technique is explained and illustrated in chapter 9 on page 109.

| Table 3.3 | Adaptations for different room temperatures | |
|---|---|
| **Adaptations for a cold room** | **Adaptations for a warm room** |
| Longer and more active warm-up. | Shorter and less intense warm-up. |
| More pulse-raising moves between stretches. | Safer to perform more static stretches. |
| Longer and more intense cardio-vascular activities. | Less intense, and perhaps slightly shorter duration, cardio-vascular activities. |
| Less time on muscular strength and endurance activities; too many have a cooling effect on the body, so you may need to prioritise muscles. | More time on muscular strength and endurance activities to replace cardio-vascular work. |
| Shorter post-workout stretch; perhaps combine stretches to save time and leave out, or prioritise, developmental stretches (perform maintenance stretches instead). | Longer post-workout stretch; include more developmental stretches and hold for longer. |
| Leave out relaxation techniques. | Longer relaxation component. |
| Longer to re-warm and re-mobilise. | Shorter re-mobilise. |

## What are the safety considerations regarding attire for an ETM session?

### Footwear

There is a whole range of different footwear available for exercise and fitness activities. Most sports companies design specific footwear for each specific sport and activity. Participants should seek advice from either the sales staff in a sports shop or from the manufacturer before deciding on the appropriate type. As a guide, the footwear selected should be well fitting, supportive and designed specifically for the type of activity for which it is to be used. Participants who take part in a number of different activities are wise to invest in cross trainers, which are designed for use in a variety of sports. Active exercisers should also replace their footwear regularly. Constant use creates wear and tear on the shoes so they become less supportive over an extended period of time. Ideally, footwear should be used exclusively for sporting activities and not for everyday use as this will increase their longevity.

### Clothing

All clothing should be close fitted but not so tight that movement is restricted. The disadvantage of wearing baggy clothing is that observation of joint alignment is restricted. This makes it difficult for the teacher to correct technique. However, some participants may prefer to wear a T-shirt and tracksuit bottoms as opposed to a fitted leotard and if this is their preference it should be accommodated. The main consideration is that the teacher wears clothing that allows their body alignment to be fully visible so participants can copy accurately the movement being performed. Plastic trousers should not be worn when performing high-intensity activities. They prevent the body from cooling down effectively and may cause overheating and fainting.

## Jewellery

All large items of jewellery, such as rings, bracelets, bangles, earrings and necklaces, should be removed before taking part in any physical activity. They may cause accidental injury to another participant and may become damaged or scratched during floor work or when using hand weights.

## Summary

The safety considerations discussed in this chapter are only a few of the many issues which need to be considered prior to planning an ETM session. Each sports club and dance studio will have its own rules and regulations that teachers will need to adhere and ascribe to so it is essential that the teacher becomes familiar with the requirements of the centre at which they teach. Combined efforts from all people involved will ensure that the sessions programmed are safe, effective and comply with all current health and safety legislation.

# SELECTING A PROGRAMME FORMAT

## What type of programme is suitable for the general population?

For most participants a programme that targets all the components of physical fitness will be most appropriate. Training in all the components provides a holistic approach to fitness and should satisfy most personal fitness goals and requirements. Most general ETM sessions follow the structure outlined in table 4.1, which includes effective training in all components.

The general ETM training programme is also used to specifically train for cardio-vascular fitness. Chapter 7 outlines how to design a cardio-vascular training programme based on the structure outlined in table 4.1.

There are a variety of more specific ETM programmes available that target only one or two of the components of fitness. Some target groups will require more specific ETM programmes to complement other training programmes. For example, people who run regularly may prefer to attend a sculpt class which focuses on improving their upper body strength and endurance and contains no specific cardio-vascular training. Alternatively, people who regularly work out with weights may prefer to attend a hi-lo class which focuses on improving cardio-vascular fitness and contains no specific muscular strength and endurance work. Some people may prefer to attend a stretch and relax class which focuses on improving their flexibility and relaxing their mind and body.

Employers and aerobic co-ordinators are always looking for new approaches to ETM to expand their existing timetable, so it is beneficial for ETM teachers to become aware of the variety of programmes that exist and alternative approaches that can be adopted.

| Table 4.1 | The general ETM programme structure | |
|---|---|---|
| Programme | Session structure | Fitness component |
| General ETM | Warm-up component | Preparation of the body systems |
| | Main workout (part 1): cardio-vascular training | Cardio-vascular fitness |
| | Main workout (part 2) muscular strength and endurance training | Muscular strength and muscular endurance |
| | Cool-down component | Flexibility (if developmental stretches are included in cool-down) |

## What types of programmes are available?

There are a variety of different types of programmes that can each be designed to train one or more of the specific components of fitness. An outline of some of the different approaches to ETM that can be implemented are detailed in table 4.2. However, the programmes are not a definitive list: there are endless ways to vary each of the sessions and create a whole new programme. The key principle is that the programme implemented meets the personal fitness goals of the participants and is appropriate for the environment. For all the programmes listed, the main workout should be preceded and concluded by a thorough and appropriate warm-up and cool-down.

| Table 4.2 | Alternative approaches to ETM | |
|---|---|---|
| Programme | Session structure | Fitness components trained in the main workout |
| Circuit | Warm-up component | Preparation of the body systems |
| | Main workout: circuit training | Cardio-vascular fitness and muscular strength and endurance |
| | Cool-down component | Flexibility (by including developmental post-workout stretches in the cool-down) |
| Step | Warm-up component | Preparation of the body systems |
| | Main workout: step training | Cardio-vascular fitness and muscular endurance for the lower body |
| | Cool-down component | Flexibility (by including developmental post-workout stretches in the cool-down) |
| | Note: a variation can be to follow the general session structure and include two main workouts to cover all components. | Note: participants should be advised to to include upper body muscular strength strength and endurance training in their other weekly training sessions to provide muscle balance. |
| Resistance (Body conditioning, Body Sculpt, New Body etc.) | Warm-up component | Preparation of the body systems |
| | Main workout: resistance training | Muscular strength and muscular endurance (whole body approach) |
| | Cool-down component | Flexibility (if developmental stretches are included in post-workout stretch) |

| Table 4.2 | Alternative approaches to ETM cont. | |
|---|---|---|
| Programme | Session structure | Fitness components trained in the main workout |
| Stretch and relax | Warm-up component | Preparation of the body systems |
| | Main workout: flexibility | Flexibility (developmental stretches) |
| | Cool-down component | Flexibility (developmental stretches) |
| | | Note: warming movements need to be maintained throughout this type of class to ensure that muscles are sufficiently warm for stretching |

*Note*: careful consideration should be given to the structure, design and content of any of these training programmes to ensure they assist in achieving participants' personal fitness goals and are safe to perform in the studio environment. A stretch class will not be safe to perform in a cold room.

Some of the alternative approaches to ETM are explained in detail in section three of this book. Each chapter in section three explains how to structure the specific components and illustrates some appropriate exercises. The exercises selected focus primarily on training healthy individuals without specialist requirements, however most of the exercises can be adapted to suit specialist groups. This can be achieved by varying their intensity and guidelines are provided on how to progress and adapt each exercise to cater for different groups.

warming up before the main workout commences, and for cooling down afterwards. It is also essential that the timing and intensity of the exercises selected for the main workout reflect the requirements of the target group. Specific guidelines for the content of each component of the session are explained and illustrated through all chapters in section three.

## How should an ETM programme be structured?

All ETM sessions must be structured safely and effectively to maximise the benefits of the activity and reduce the risk of injury. It is essential that appropriate time is allocated for

| Table 4.3 | An outline of the duration and intensity of components for different target groups | | |
|---|---|---|---|
| | *Less fit and specialist groups* | *Intermediate fitness level and general groups* | *Advanced fitness level and sport-specific groups* |
| Overall duration | 45 minutes | 45–60 minutes | 60 minutes |
| Overall intensity of session components | Low | Moderate | High |
| Speed of movements | Slow pace | Moderate pace | Fast pace |
| Warm-up component (mobility, pulse-raising, preparatory stretch) | Long duration and low intensity<br><br>15–20 minutes | Moderate duration and intensity<br><br>10–15 minutes | Short duration and high intensity<br><br>10–15 minutes |
| Main workout (1): cardio-vascular training (re-warm, maintain, pulse lower) | Short duration and low intensity<br><br>10–15 minutes | Moderate duration and intensity<br><br>20 minutes | Long duration and high intensity<br><br>20–30 minutes |
| Main workout (2): muscular strength and endurance training | Moderate duration and low intensity<br><br>10–12 minutes | Moderate duration and intensity<br><br>10–12 minutes | Long duration and high intensity<br><br>10–20 minutes |
| Cool-down component (developmental and maintenance post-workout stretches, relaxation, re-mobilise) | Long duration and low intensity<br><br>10–13 minutes | Moderate duration and intensity<br><br>5–10 minutes | Short duration and high intensity<br><br>5–10 minutes |

*Note*: these timings are only guidelines and are variable depending on the environment, the requirements of the individual/group and the structure of the main workout.

# DESIGNING A WARM-UP

5

## Why do we need to warm up before the main workout?

We need to warm up prior to activity to prepare all the bodily systems for the activity that will follow. Warming up will potentially enhance our performance and may reduce the risk of injury. A thorough warm-up should therefore help to maximise the safety and effectiveness of the activity. It is therefore essential that appropriate time is set aside for warming up before the main workout commences. It is also essential that the correct exercises are selected. This chapter discusses what should happen to the body during this preparatory component of the session (the short-term physiological responses). It also outlines how to design a safe and effective warm-up and achieve the desired responses.

## What types of exercises should the warm-up contain?

The warm-up needs to prepare the joints, muscles, heart, circulatory and neuromuscular systems for the main workout. It should contain exercises that achieve the desired effects outlined in table 5.1.

| Table 5.1 | The desired effects of the warm-up on the body |
|---|---|

Warm-up exercises should be characterised by the following.

- They should promote the release of synovial fluid into the joint capsule and warm the tendons, muscles and ligaments which surround each joint. This will ensure the joints are adequately lubricated and cushioned, and will allow a fuller range of motion to be achieved at each joint. This can be achieved by **mobility exercises**.
- They should increase the heart rate, promote an increase of blood flow to the muscles and an increase in the delivery of oxygen. This will make the body warmer, the muscles more pliable and will allow them to work more comfortably throughout the main workout. This can be achieved by **pulse-raising exercises**.
- They should lengthen the muscles and move them through a larger range of motion. This may lower the risk of injury if moving into extended positions in the main workout. This can be achieved by **stretching exercises**.
- They should activate the brain and neuro-muscular pathways, focusing attention and concentration by rehearsing skills and move-ment patterns, rehearsing the muscle and joint actions in the way they are to be moved in the main workout, and raising the heart rate to a desired training level. This can be achieved by **re-warming exercises**.

## What types of exercises are appropriate to mobilise the joints?

Moving each of the joint areas through its natural range of motion will achieve the desired effects listed in table 5.1. All of the joints to be used in the main workout should be targeted. Examples of the main actions of the joints and appropriate exercises for mobilising each joint area are outlined in table 5.2. The exercises selected should start with a small range of motion and progressively move to a larger range of motion. However, they should only be taken through a range of motion that is comfortable for the individual to achieve.

An example of progressively building the range of motion for the shoulder joint is to start with lifting and lowering the shoulders (elevation and depression), progress to rolling and rotating the shoulders, and finish by performing the larger movements such as taking the arms to the side of the body and back in (abduction and adduction), and fully circling the arm (circumduction). It should be noted that this is not intended to be the definitive guide on how to warm up this joint area; it is simply an example of how the range of motion can be progressed in one joint area.

Exercises to mobilise the joints are illustrated with step-by-step instructions later in this chapter (*see* pages 47–53).

## Which joints need to be mobilised?

The main selection of mobility exercises should focus on preparing the specific joints that will be doing the majority of the work planned for the main session. The primary focus for a cardio-vascular training session should be the lower body because the joints in this area will need to cushion the impact force and support most of the body weight during the main workout. The arms will also be used to some extent and therefore a little mobility work for the upper body is always advisable.

Alternatively, if the main workout is a body conditioning, toning or sculpting class, the upper body will be trained more. Resistance equipment such as bands, barbells or dumbbells may also be used. If this is the case, it is advisable to prioritise the upper body joints, since they will be bearing a lot more weight throughout the session.

Ideally, the warm-up should be planned after the main session activities to ensure that the body is appropriately prepared. It is neither safe nor effective to prepare only the upper body, when in fact the lower body is doing a large proportion of the work in the main session. Ultimately, it is advisable to prepare all the joints, since it is likely that all joint areas will receive work during the main session.

## How will mobility exercises alter for different groups?

The range of motion that we have at each joint can vary from one joint area to another. It can also vary from one individual to another. The starting point of the first mobility exercise will depend on the range of motion capabilities in the group.

Newcomers to ETM will need to start with a small range of motion and may not be able to build up to a very large range of motion. The movements may also need to be performed at a slightly slower pace and with more emphasis on control. It may also be advisable to perform more repetitions, or sets of repetitions, of the same exercises for beginners to achieve the desired mobility effects.

A fitter group may be able to safely start with a large range of motion and should be able to progress to a much fuller range of motion without any discomfort. They should also be

| Table 5.2 | The actions possible at each joint and appropriate exercises to achieve that action | |
|---|---|---|
| Joint area | Joint actions possible | Appropriate exercises |
| Ankle | Plantarflexion and dorsiflexion | Heel and toe alternately pointing to the floor (see page 53) Walking/pedalling through the feet Rotating/circling the foot |
| Knee | Flexion and extension | Bending and straightening the knees (Squats) Kicking the heel to the bottom (Leg Curls, see page 51) |
| Hip | Flexion and extension | Lifting the knees up towards the chest and down again Lunging the leg backwards and forwards (Back Lunges) |
| | Abduction and adduction | Taking the leg out to the side and back in (low-impact Jumping Jacks) |
| | Rotation | Mambos involve some rotation of the hip |
| Spine | Lateral flexion and extension Rotation Flexion and extension | Side Bends (see page 48) Side Twists (see page 49) Humping and hollowing the spine (see page 50) |
| Shoulder and shoulder girdle | Elevation and depression | Lifting and lowering the shoulders (see page 47) |
| | Abduction and adduction | Taking the arms out to the side of the body and back in |
| | Rotation | Rotating the arm in a figure-of-eight motion towards and away from the body |
| | Horizontal flexion and extension | With the arms at shoulder level bring the arms across the front of the body and back to start position (Pec Decs) |
| | Circumduction | Moving the arm in a complete circle |
| Elbow | Flexion, extension and rotation | Bending and straightening the elbow |

able to work through to their full range of motion at a slightly faster pace, with fewer sets of repetitions for specific joint areas. They should be able to warm up their joints more quickly due to their increased body awareness and more effective physiological responses to warm-up activities. However, it is essential, even with fitter groups, that the movements do not become too energetic and too large until the muscles are really warm. There will be a greater risk of damaging the tissues that surround the joints (muscles, tendons and ligaments) if the range of motion is built up too quickly.

## What types of exercises are appropriate to raise the pulse?

Rhythmic movements that utilise the larger lower body muscle groups will achieve the desired effects outlined in table 5.1. Movement of the legs will progressively increase the heart rate and blood flow through the muscles. This will ensure that adequate oxygen is delivered to the muscles, which will be needed to fuel their activities through the main session. It will also ensure the muscles are sufficiently warm and safe to stretch. The arms are less effective at raising the heart rate and getting the body warm. This is because the muscles are smaller and do not demand large volumes of oxygen to be delivered. However, they are used to create variety and develop motor skills.

There are a whole variety of movements that are effective in warming the muscles and increasing the heart rate. Marching, Leg Curls, Squats and walking forwards and backwards, to name a few, are all very effective. These exercises are low impact and put little stress on the joints. High-impact exercises will often place great stress on the joints, and may raise the intensity too quickly, so they are best saved for the main cardio-vascular workout. It is impor-

tant that the exercises selected do not become too intense for the body to cope with at this early stage in the session. Ultimately, the level of intensity and impact of exercises will be dependent on the fitness level and individual requirements of the individuals performing them.

It is just as important that the pulse-raising movements selected make gradual demands on the body. They too should start at a relatively low intensity and progress to a moderate intensity. This can be achieved by starting out with a basic movement, such as a Squat, without bending deeply. To build the intensity the bend can become deeper, the Squats can be travelled to the right or left, and the arms can be used to add variety and create a little more momentum. Once again the speed of the progression from one stage to another, and the starting level of intensity, depends on the fitness level of the group.

Pulse-raising exercises are illustrated with step-by-step illustrations later in this chapter (*see* pages 54–58).

## How will pulse-raising exercises alter for different groups?

Newcomers may need to start at a very low level of intensity. They will not need to, or be able to, progress to a high level of intensity to get warm. Low levels of intensity can be achieved by working with shallower bends, lower impact exercises, smaller ranges of motion, comparatively less travel and slower pace.

Fitter groups can start at a moderate level of intensity and finish at a much higher level of intensity. Higher levels of intensity can be achieved by working through a larger range of motion, bending deeper, moving at a slightly faster pace and travelling more. It is worth noting for all fitness levels that if the warm-up or pulse-raising activities start at too high an intensity, the muscles may undergo an oxygen deficit (they will not be supplied with sufficient oxygen) and if this occurs they will tire very quickly and will not be able to work effectively through the main session. This reinforces the need for the warm-up to be gradual and progressive for all fitness levels.

## What types of exercises are appropriate to stretch the muscles?

Exercises that allow the muscles to lengthen will achieve the desired effects outlined in table 5.1. Chapter 1 details two types of stretching exercises that are appropriate for an etm session: static stretches and moving stretches. Static stretches are those where the muscle is lengthened to a point where mild tension is experienced, and then held still until the tension subsides; moving stretches are those where the muscle is lengthened and moved slowly to a point where a mild tension is felt, and then returned back to its normal starting position. This process is generally repeated a few times so that each time the muscle eases slightly further into an extended position.

Static stretches are generally much safer because they allow a slower and more gradual movement into the stretch position and participants are less likely to overstretch. However, a routine that only includes static stretches will tend to allow the body to cool down too much and the benefits of the warm-up may be lost. If static stretches are preferred, a larger proportion of pulse-raising movements performed between stretches will be necessary to keep the body warm. This will, however, depend on the temperature of the room. In warmer weather and when working in a warmer room, the body will not cool down as much. In these circumstances it is perfectly acceptable to

perform a higher proportion of static stretches, and a lower proportion of pulse-raising movements between stretches. One should remember, though, that if the muscles are allowed to cool down then they will no longer stretch so effectively. Stretching cold muscles could also potentially cause them injury.

Moving stretches are becoming increasingly popular, but great care should be taken to ensure that participants do not exceed a comfortable range of motion and do not move into the stretch too quickly – the speed at which moving stretches are performed is crucial to their safety. If the music used is too quick and the stretch position is moved into too quickly, the stretch may be performed ballistically, which may cause damage and tearing of the muscles. It is more appropriate to use moving stretches with individuals with good skills and body awareness; it is also advisable to perform a static stretch of the muscle before performing a moving stretch. This will at least allow the muscle sufficient time to relax and lengthen.

Preparatory stretches are illustrated with step-by-step instructions later in this chapter (*see* pages 59–66). The floor-based post-workout stretches illustrated in chapter 6 (*see* pages 72–80) may also be used in a warm-up.

## Which muscles need to be stretched?

All the muscles to be used in the main session should be lengthened prior to work. Priority should be given to those muscles that will be working the hardest. If the main session is to consist of a large proportion of cardio-vascular exercises, or lower body resistance exercises, the muscles of the lower body are a priority. Alternatively, a muscular strength and endurance (conditioning and sculpting) workout, which specifically targets the upper body, will require a greater focus on stretching the muscles of the upper body and trunk.

Overall, it is advisable to stretch all the muscles, since it is unlikely that a specific body area will not be used at all in the session. A range of appropriate stretches for each specific muscle group is illustrated at the end of this chapter.

## How will stretching exercises alter for different groups?

The type of stretch selected will be determined by the ability of the participants. Static stretches are potentially safer for those with low skill levels and a small range of movement because a safe range of motion is less likely to be exceeded when holding stretches in a static position. This is, of course, provided that the range of motion has not already been exceeded. If more than a mild tension is experienced, or if the muscle begins to shake, it is a sure sign that the stretch has been taken too far. If this is the case, it is advisable to reduce the range of motion slightly or move out of the stretch and try again, this time moving into the stretch position more carefully.

Moving stretches require greater body awareness to prevent a safe range of motion being exceeded. They are more appropriate for individuals who are experienced, have greater body awareness, and for those with a large range of movement.

## What is the purpose of re-warming?

Since the body may have cooled down slightly after performing the preparatory stretches, it is essential to re-warm the muscles before commencing the main workout. In addition, the re-warmer can be used to prepare the body specifically for the main workout. It allows a rehearsal of specific movement patterns to occur that will stimulate the neuromuscular pathways. This will help to improve the performance of all movements and enhance the effectiveness of the main workout. In a training session which includes cardio-vascular work the re-warmer should build the heart rate into the aerobic training zone. This is sometimes referred to as build-up aerobics and forms the first part of the cardio-vascular component.

## What types of exercises are appropriate for re-warming the body?

The movements to be used in the main workout are appropriate for re-warming. However, it is essential that the intensity of the movements starts at a relatively low pace and builds up progressively to the level of intensity required for the main workout. This is to maximise use of the aerobic energy system and avoid unnecessary discomfort which may be experienced from using anaerobic energy systems as the primary fuel for movement. The latter is more likely to occur if the intensity starts too high or builds up too quickly. Ultimately, the intensity of the exercises will depend on the fitness level of the individuals, and the activities used within the main workout.

## How will the main workout affect the exercises selected for the re-warmer?

If the main workout is to consist solely or predominantly of resistance training exercises (muscular strength and endurance), the exercises selected for the re-warmer should resemble the movements to be used, but at a slightly lower intensity. For example, if weights are to be used, an initial set of the main workout exercises performed with a lower weight is probably adequate to re-warm and prepare the muscles. It may also be necessary to incorporate some larger pulse-raising movements throughout this component of a resistance training session to ensure the body does not cool down and a comfortable body temperature is maintained.

In a training session that includes cardio-vascular work, the re-warmer should raise the heart rate to the aerobic training zone. This part of the warm-up is sometimes referred to as build-up aerobics and becomes part of the main workout for specific cardio-vascular training sessions. These sessions may be included in either a general (*see* chapter 7), step (*see* chapter 8) or circuit training (*see* chapter 10) programme.

If the main workout is to comprise solely of cardio-vascular or aerobic training exercises, the movements in the re-warmer should resemble less energetic versions of those to be used in the main session. The exercises should start at a less energetic pace and progressively build up to a higher level of intensity. For example, a Jumping Jack can start without the jump by stepping alternate legs out to the side. This can progress by bending deeper, adding arms for momentum, adding a small hop between lunges, and can finish by jumping both legs out to the side. The exercise can be progressed even further by performing a Power Jack and/or travelling the movement. In practice, it is advisable for a sequence of movements to be selected and repeated three or four times, each time making each of the movements a little harder. This will progressively raise the intensity.

## How will the re-warmer alter for different groups?

Newcomers to etm will need to start at a low level of intensity. They will need to spend slightly longer building up the range of motion to ensure the intensity is raised at a gradual pace and their body is able to cope with the demands being made upon it.

A fitter group can start at a higher intensity and can work hard much sooner. They should not need to spend so long on this specific component. They can still work progressively to a higher level, but will be able to move to a higher intensity much sooner because their cardio-vascular system will deliver and utilise the oxygen they demand more effectively.

## What factors affect the overall timing and intensity of the warm-up?

- Room and external temperature.
- Fitness level.
- Age of participants.

The temperature of the room and the external temperature will affect the duration and intensity of the warm-up. First, it will determine the starting point for the range of motion of mobility exercises. The muscles and other tissues that surround the joints are less pliable when they are cold, so attempting to move the joint areas through too large a range of motion before they are sufficiently warm will increase the risk of injury to these tissues. In a cold room, it is advisable to commence with some gentle pulse-raising movements to get the body warm before moving the joints through too large a range of motion, and to spend a longer time keeping the body warm between stretches. The increased amount of pulse-raising neces-sary will therefore require a longer warm-up.

In a warm room and on a warm day the joints can be moved to a fuller range of motion sooner. It will be safer to perform joint mobility exercises before any specific pulse-raising activities, and to perform a higher number of static stretches with less pulse-raising moves. Therefore, the warm-up can be shorter when the room is warm.

Newcomers and specialist groups need a longer warm-up with a more gradual progression of intensity to ensure the demands made upon the body do not create an oxygen deficit. Specific adaptations to adjust the intensity of each individual stage of the warm-up to accommodate different fitness levels is discussed earlier in this chapter.

## How should the warm-up be structured for an etm session?

The warm-up should be structured in three stages:

1 mobility and pulse-raising exercises (general warm-up)
2 preparatory stretches
3 re-warmer (specific warm-up).

## What is the appropriate posture to maintain when performing warm-up exercises?

An appropriate posture to maintain while performing all of the exercises illustrated in this book is outlined below.

- Abdominal muscles pulled in to maintain a fixed position of the lower spine.
- Spine long and upright.
- Shoulders relaxed and down.
- Back straight.
- Head up.
- Bottom tucked under.
- Knees unlocked.

### Summary of the guidelines for planning the warm-up

- Start with small mobility and pulse-raising exercises and gradually build up the range of motion and intensity of the movements. This can be achieved by progressively moving through a larger range of motion, bending deeper, travelling more and moving at a progressively faster pace.
- Combine static mobility exercises with larger pulse-raising movements for groups with greater skill to create interest and maintain the pace of the warm-up.
- Use low-impact pulse-raising moves since these are less stressful for the body.
- Ensure that the body is completely warm before stretching and moving to a larger range of motion.
- Combine static stretches with larger pulse-raising moves to maintain the pace of the warm-up and prevent the body from cooling down.

# MOBILITY AND/OR PULSE-RAISING EXERCISES

| **Ex 1** | **Shoulder lifts and rolls (mobility)** |
|---|---|

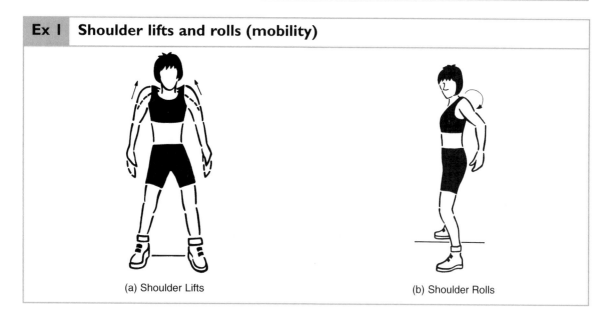

(a) Shoulder Lifts

(b) Shoulder Rolls

## Purpose

These exercises mobilise the shoulder joint and can be performed with the pulse-raising exercises for variety if participants have sufficient motor skills.

## Starting position and instructions

Start with the feet hip width apart and (a) lift alternate shoulders towards the ears or both shoulders together; (b) roll alternate shoulders backwards or roll both shoulders together. These exercises can be performed with a step and tap movement where the body weight is shifted from one side to the other. Continue for the desired number of repetitions.

## Teaching points

- Maintain an upright posture with the back straight and chest lifted.
- Keep the hips facing forwards and tighten the abdominal muscles.
- Keep the knee joints unlocked.
- Move the shoulders at a controlled speed and progressively aim to move in a larger range of motion.

## Progressions

- Start with a small range of motion and progressively increase the range.
- Move at a progressively faster tempo.
- Use longer levers by moving the elbow around or the full arm around for shoulder rolls.
- Vary the speed and/or combine the movements together, for example lift the shoulders together slowly doing two repetitions for eight counts, and then alternate shoulder rolls at a quicker pace for eight counts.
- Combine the shoulder mobility exercises with other mobility exercises or pulse-raising exercises to increase the skill level.
- Add variety by rolling the elbows back and combing the fingers through the hair.

| Ex 2 | Side bends (mobility) |
|---|---|

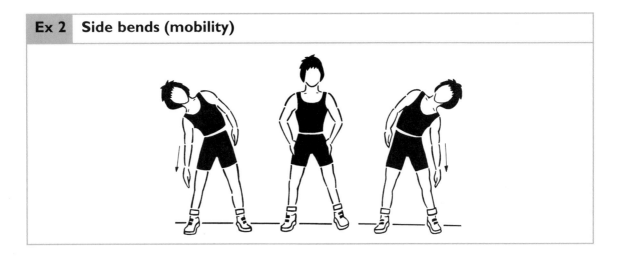

## Purpose

This exercise will mobilise the thoracic vertebrae of the spine.

## Starting position and instructions

Start with the feet hip width apart, the body upright and the knees unlocked. Bend directly to the right side in a controlled manner. Return to the upright position. Bend directly to the left side in a controlled manner. Return to the upright position. Continue for the desired number of repetitions.

## Teaching points

- Bend only as far as is comfortable.
- Keep the hips facing forwards and avoid hollowing of the lower back by tightening the abdominal muscles.
- Keep the movement controlled.
- Keep the body lifted between the hips and the ribs.
- Lift up before bending to the side.
- Lean directly to the side and ensure the body does not roll forwards or backwards.
- Visualise your body as being placed between two panes of glass.

## Progressions

- Start with a small bend and progress to a slightly larger range of motion, but only as far as is comfortable.
- Start by alternating the bending movement from right to left and progress by performing more repetitions to one side before changing sides. This will require slightly greater muscular endurance to maintain correct alignment.
- Move at a slightly faster pace by increasing the speed of the music. Take care not to move too fast and create excessive momentum as this may cause the movement to become ballistic.
- Travel a greater distance by increasing the number of repetitions in one direction.
- Vary the speed by performing one slow side bend in each direction (down and up to centre, down and up to centre – eight counts total), and then perform four quick single bends without the pause at the central position. This will require greater skill from participants.
- Perform a shoulder shrug or two alternate shoulder lifts in between each side bend when the spine is aligned centrally. This will require greater motor skills and will save time spent on the overall warm-up as the shoulder joints are also mobilised.

## Ex 3   Side twists (spine mobility)

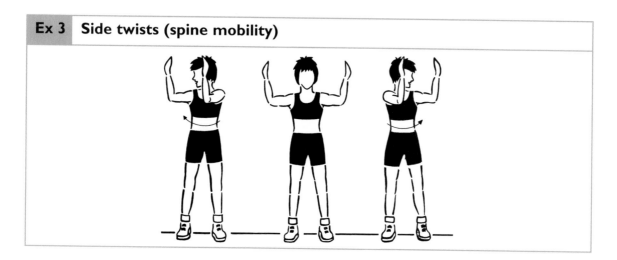

### Purpose

This exercise will mobilise the thoracic vertebrae of the spine.

### Starting position and instructions

Start with the feet a shoulder width and a half apart. Hold the arms at shoulder level with the elbows slightly bent. Twist around to one side, return to the centre and then twist to the other side.

### Teaching points

- Keep the hips and knees facing forwards, do not let the knee joints roll inwards.
- Keep the knees slightly bent.
- Make sure the lower back does not twist.
- Keep the abdominals pulled in, the chest lifted, shoulders relaxed and back straight.

### Progressions

- Start slow and work through a small range of motion.
- Increase progressively the speed of the movement and move through a slightly larger range of motion. Note: ensure that the speed of movement remains appropriately controlled and that the range of motion allows for correct spinal alignment to be maintained.
- Keep the hands on the hips instead of held high to take out any fixator work of the deltoid (shoulder) muscles.

## Ex 4 | Hump and straighten (spine mobility)

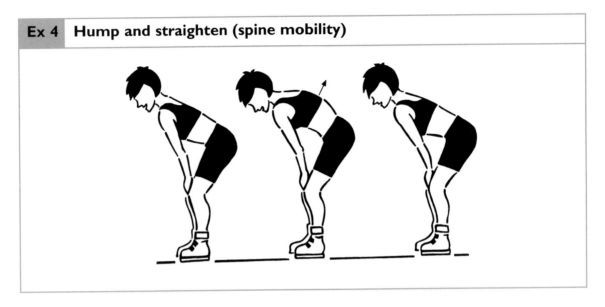

*Note*: ensure the body is adequately warmed up before moving to a more extended position.

### Purpose

This exercise will mobilise the lumbar vertebrae of the spine.

### Starting position and instructions

Start with the feet a shoulder width and a half apart and the knees slightly bent. Lean the body forwards and place the hands on the knees. Round the back, i.e. hump the spine. Release by returning the back to a flattened position.

### Teaching points

- Keep the hips and knees facing forwards, do not let the knee joints roll inwards.
- Keep the knees slightly bent.
- Make sure the lower back does not hollow or twist.
- Keep the body weight supported throughout the movement.
- Keep the abdominals pulled in, the chest lifted and shoulders relaxed.

### Progressions

- Start by standing upright and just rounding the shoulders and upper back forwards and backwards.
- Start slow and work through a small range of motion.
- Progressively increase the speed of the movement and move through a slightly larger range of motion. Note: ensure that the speed of movement remains appropriately controlled and that the range of motion allows for correct spinal alignment to be maintained.
- As a variation, press alternate shoulders forwards, i.e. right shoulder to left knee and left shoulder to right knee, but take care not to hollow the spine or twist too far and too quickly.

## Ex 5    Leg curls (mobility)

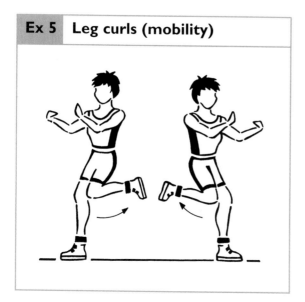

### Purpose

This exercise assists primarily with mobilising the knee joints. It will also assist with raising the pulse and warming the muscles since the muscles of the legs will be weight bearing when transferring the weight of the body from one side to the other. If it is performed with a greater intensity or with impact, it can be used effectively to improve cardio-vascular fitness.

### Starting position and instructions

Start with the feet hip width apart. Step out to the right and transfer the weight over to the right, kicking the left heel towards the buttocks. Step the left leg down and transfer the weight over to the left leg, kicking the right heel to the buttocks. Continue alternating the Leg Curls for the desired number of repetitions.

### Teaching points

- Take a large, but comfortable, stride.
- Keep the hips facing forwards and avoid hollowing of the lower back by tightening the abdominal muscles.
- Ensure the knee joint remains unlocked when landing.
- Ensure the knees move in line with the toes and do not roll inwards.
- Keep the back straight and the chest lifted.
- Keep the movement controlled and smooth.
- If the exercise is used for cardio-vascular training and impact is added, make sure the heels go down to cushion the movement.

### Progressions

- Start with a small stride and progressively increase stride length, but ensure the distance is comfortable and correct alignment is maintained.
- Move at a progressively faster pace.
- Bend deeper to promote greater pulse-raising.
- Travel the movement forwards and backwards: this will add intensity because the body weight is being shifted across gravity. Progress further by travelling a greater distance in each direction.
- Perform two or more leg curls to the same side. This requires slightly greater muscular endurance and will vary the choreography.
- Add a turn to the movement, for example: face front and step right, kicking the left heel up to the bottom, quarter turning the body to the right as the left leg comes down; face right and kick the right heel to the bottom and return to face front as the left leg kicks the bottom; face front and kick the right leg to the bottom, quarter turning to the left as the right leg lowers down; face left and kick the left heel to the bottom and return to face front as the right leg kicks the bottom.

## Ex 6  Knee lifts (mobility)

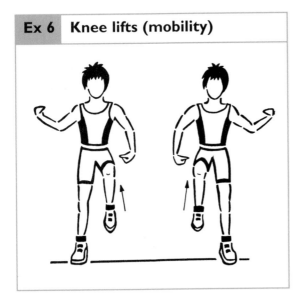

## Purpose

This exercise mobilises the hip joint. It will assist with raising the pulse and warming the muscles because the legs are bearing the body weight throughout the movement. If it is performed with greater intensity, or with impact, it can be used effectively to improve cardio-vascular fitness.

## Starting position and instructions

Start with the feet hip width apart. Step and shift the weight on to the right leg, lifting the left knee to hip height. Step and shift the weight on to the left leg, lifting the right knee to hip height. Continue to alternate knee raises for the desired number of repetitions.

## Teaching points

- Take a comfortable stride of the legs.
- Keep the hips facing forwards and avoid hollowing of the lower back by tightening the abdominal muscles.
- Keep the knee joints unlocked and ensure the knees stay in line with the toes.

- Lift the leg only to a height where an upright spinal alignment can be maintained.
- Keep the chest lifted and do not allow the body to bend forwards as the leg lifts.
- If the exercise is used for cardio-vascular training and impact is added, make sure the heels go down to cushion the movement.

## Progressions

- Start by lifting the leg only to a small height and progressively lift the leg higher.
- Bend the weight-bearing leg more to add intensity.
- Move at a slightly faster pace.
- Turn the movement in a circle (or as described for Leg Curls, see exercise 5, progressions) to add variety and challenge motor skills.
- Perform two or more repetitions on the same side. This requires greater muscular endurance.
- Travel the movement forwards and backwards to achieve a greater pulse-raising effect. Increase this further by travelling a greater distance and increasing the number of repetitions in one direction.
- For cardio-vascular training, add impact to shift the resistance of the body upwards against gravity and to increase intensity.
- To add further intensity for cardio-vascular training, perform four or more repetitions on each side and travel the movement in the direction of the knee that is lifting.

## Ex 7 | Heel and toe (mobility)

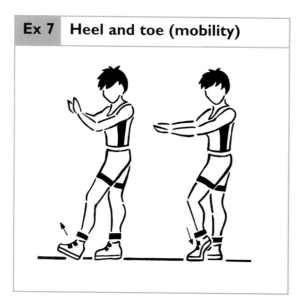

## Purpose

This exercise mobilises the ankle joint. If performed with the weight-bearing leg hopping it can be used as a cardio-vascular exercise.

## Starting position and instructions

Start with the feet hip width apart and take the weight on to one leg. Dig the heel of the other foot towards the floor and then point the toe towards the floor. Continue for the desired number of repetitions and perform on the other leg.

## Teaching points

- Keep the weight-bearing leg soft and do not allow the knee to roll in.
- Keep the hips facing forwards and the back straight.
- Keep the movement controlled.
- Keep the knee joints unlocked and ensure the knees move in line with the toes.
- Aim for the heel and toe to land in the same place to ensure a full range of motion of the ankle is achieved.
- For cardio-vascular work, if impact is added, make sure the heels go down to cushion the movement.

## Progressions

- Start with a small range of motion and progress to a large range of motion.
- Move progressively to a faster pace.
- Reduce the repetitions on each side to increase motor skills.
- Increase the repetitions on each side to increase muscular endurance.
- Add upper body movement to add motor skills.
- Circle the ankle as a variation.
- Bend and straighten the weight-bearing leg to add motor skills and to maintain the tempo of the session.

## Ex 8 Scoops (pulse-raising)

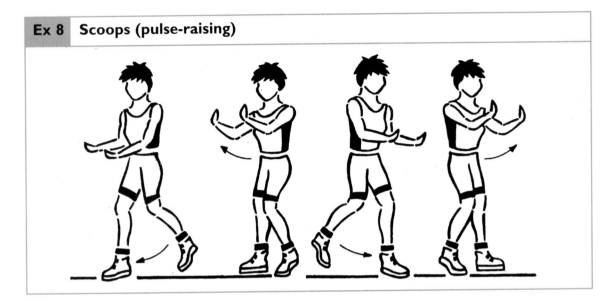

## Purpose

This exercise assists primarily with raising the pulse and warming the muscles. If it is performed with greater intensity, or with impact, it can be used effectively to improve cardio-vascular fitness.

## Starting position and instructions

Start with the feet hip width apart. Step diagonally forwards to the right corner leading with the right leg. Draw the left leg in to meet the right, simultaneously making scooping actions with the arms. Step diagonally forwards to the left side with the left leg leading. Continue alternating diagonal scoops for the desired number of repetitions.

## Teaching points

- Take a large, but comfortable, stride.
- Keep the hips facing forwards and avoid hollowing of the lower back by tightening the abdominal muscles.
- Keep movements of the shoulder joints controlled.
- Keep the knee joints unlocked and ensure the knees move in line with the toes.
- If impact is added, make sure the heels go down to cushion the movement.

## Progressions

- Start with a small stride and progressively increase stride length.
- Move at a progressively faster pace.
- Travel a greater distance by increasing the number of repetitions in one direction.
- Perform two or more scoops in the same direction to vary choreography.
- Add impact and jump higher to shift the resistance of the body upwards and against the force of gravity and to increase intensity.
- Vary the speed, i.e. perform one slow power scoop right (two counts), one slow power scoop left (two counts), then perform four quick, single count scoops.

## Ex 9 Side squats (pulse-raising)

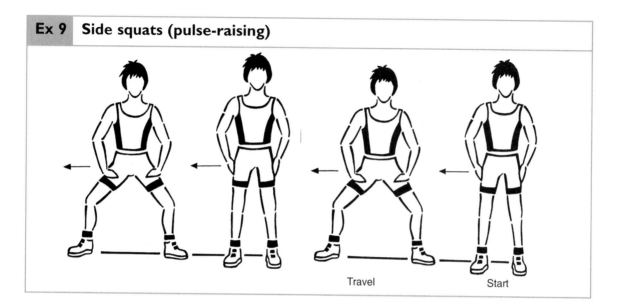

Travel      Start

## Purpose

This exercise assists primarily with raising the pulse and warming the muscles. If a reasonably wide stride is taken on the squat movement there may be some mobilisation benefits for the hip. In addition, the bending and straightening action of the knee will provide some mobilisation for this area. If the arms are used there may be some mobilisation benefits for the shoulder and elbow joint. If performed with a deeper bend and greater travel, this exercise can be used in the main workout as a low-impact exercise to improve cardio-vascular fitness.

## Starting position and instructions

Start with the feet hip width apart. Commence by stepping one leg to the side and squatting the legs apart. Straighten and bring the feet together again, travelling to the side. Continue this action in the same direction for the desired number of repetitions.

## Teaching points

- Progressively increase the range of motion of the Squat, but only move through a range of motion that feels comfortable and achievable.
- Keep the hips facing forwards and avoid hollowing of the lower back by tightening the abdominal muscles.
- Avoid locking the knees as the leg straightens.
- Keep the back straight and the chest lifted.
- Ensure the knees move in line with the toes and over the ankles.
- Take care not to squat too deeply – maintain a 90° angle at the knees.

## Progressions

- Start with a static Squat in place.
- Initially take small strides and progressively increase the stride length to increase the range of motion.
- Start slow and move progressively to a faster pace.
- Perform more Squats in one direction to increase travel.

| Ex 10 | Easy walk/box steps (pulse-raising) |
|---|---|

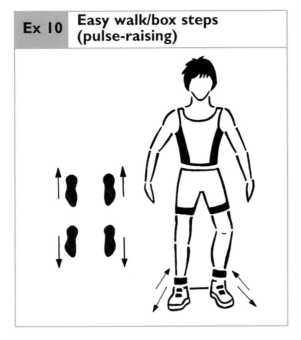

## Purpose

This exercise primarily assists with raising the pulse and warming the muscles. If it is performed with greater intensity (bending deeper), or with impact (jumping back instead of stepping back), it can be used effectively to improve cardio-vascular fitness.

## Starting position and instructions

Start with the feet hip width apart. Step forwards and take the weight on to the right leg. Step the left leg forwards so it is level with the right leg. Step the right leg backwards and take the weight on to the right leg. Step the left leg back to the start position. At this point either tap the floor with the left foot and step forwards, repeating the sequence with a left leg lead (alternating Box Step); or place the weight on to the left leg and step forwards, repeating the sequence on the right leg for the desired number of repetitions before changing legs.

## Teaching points

- Take a large, but comfortable, step forwards.
- Keep the hips facing forwards and avoid hollowing of the lower back by tightening the abdominal muscles.
- Keep the knee joints unlocked and do not allow the knees to roll inwards.
- Keep the chest lifted and body upright.
- If impact is added for cardio-vascular training, make sure the heels go down to cushion the movement.

## Progressions

- Start with a small step and progressively increase the step stride.
- Move at a progressively faster tempo.
- Bend deeper to add intensity.
- Perform more repetitions with the same leg to increase muscular endurance.
- Add impact for cardio-vascular training by either stepping forwards and jumping backwards instead of stepping backwards; or jumping forwards and stepping only on the backwards phase of the movement.

## Ex 11 Walks (pulse-raising)

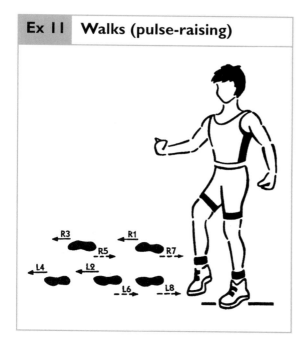

## Purpose

This exercise assists primarily with raising the pulse and warming the muscles. If it is performed with greater intensity (larger strides to travel further), or with impact (jogging instead of walking), it can be used effectively to improve cardio-vascular fitness.

## Starting position and instructions

Stand with the feet hip width apart. Walk forwards for four counts, starting with the right leg (R1, L2, R3, L4). Walk backwards for four counts (R5, L6, R7, L8).

## Teaching points

- Take a large, but comfortable, step forwards.
- Use a heel toe action when walking forwards.
- Keep the hips facing forwards and avoid hollowing of the lower back by tightening the abdominal muscles.
- Keep the knee joints unlocked and do not allow the knees to roll inwards.
- Keep the chest lifted and body upright.
- If impact is added for cardio-vascular training, make sure the heels go down to cushion the movement.

## Progressions

- Start with a small step and progressively increase the step stride.
- Move at a progressively faster tempo.
- Perform more repetitions in the same direction to assist those with limited motor skills.
- Add impact for cardio-vascular training by jogging forwards.
- Travel the movement in different directions for variation.
- Travel in a circle or figure of eight to add variety and travel further.
- Use arm lines to add variety.
- Walk with the body low ('Groucho Marx-style').

## Ex 12  Grapevines (pulse-raising)

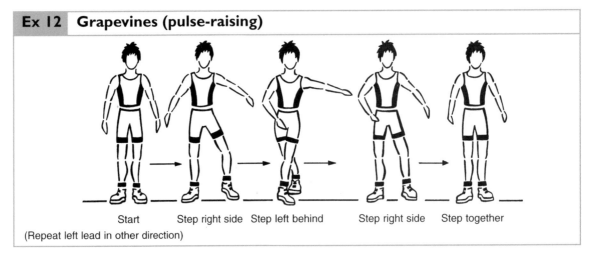

Start  Step right side Step left behind  Step right side Step together

(Repeat left lead in other direction)

### Purpose

This exercise primarily assists with raising the pulse and warming the muscles. If it is performed with greater intensity (bending deeper or travelling further), or with impact (hopping through the movement), it can effectively be used to improve cardio-vascular fitness.

### Starting position and instructions

Stand with the feet hip width apart. Step the right foot out to the right side. Cross step the left leg behind the right leg, moving the leg further in the right direction and creating a small rotation of the body. Step the right foot out to the right and place or jump the feet together. The movement can then either be repeated travelling to the right, or travelled back to the left leading with the left leg.

### Teaching points

- Take a large, but comfortable, step to the side.
- Keep the hips facing forwards and avoid hollowing of the lower back by tightening the abdominal muscles.
- Keep the knee joints slightly soft and unlocked and do not allow the knees to roll inwards.
- Keep the chest lifted and body upright.
- If impact is added for cardio-vascular training, make sure the heels go down to cushion the movement.

### Progressions

- Start with a small step and progressively increase the step stride.
- Move at a progressively faster tempo.
- Bend deeper to add intensity.
- Perform more repetitions in the same direction to increase travel and shift the centre of gravity further.
- Add impact for cardio-vascular training by either hopping through the movement or jumping at the end.
- Add a quarter turn on the jump and repeat the sequence in a box shape.
- Add a half turn on the jump and perform the left lead grapevine facing the back wall. Repeat to return to face front.
- Travel the movement forwards to the front left corner and then the front right corner, and then back to the back right corner and back left corner. Alternatively, instead of performing a grapevine back, a jump or jog back will vary choreography.
- Vary the arm lines used to add further variety.

# PREPARATORY STRETCHES

The stretches illustrated in this section include four for the lower body in standing positions, and four for the upper body, which can be performed in standing or seated positions. Floor-based stretches can also be used and these are illustrated in the section on post-workout stretches in chapter 6 (*see* pages 72–80). Likewise, these stretches can also be used for post-workout maintenance stretching.

| Ex 1 | **Back and thigh stretch** |
|---|---|

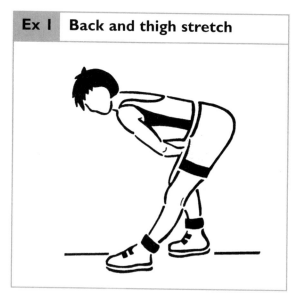

## Purpose

This exercise lengthens and stretches the hamstring muscles at the back of the thigh, and also the buttock muscles (the gluteals).

## Starting position and instructions

Stand with both feet hip width apart. Take a shoulder width stride forwards with one leg. Bend the knee of the back leg, and place the hands at the top of the thigh of the bent knee. Bend forwards from the hips and slide the hands down the thigh of the bent knee until a mild tension is felt at the back of the thigh of the straight leg. Keep the front foot flat on the ground.

## Teaching points

- Keep the weight-bearing knee joint slightly bent and ensure the knee joint does not roll inwards.
- Only bend forwards to a point where a mild tension is felt at the back of the thigh.
- Keep the knee of the straight leg fully extended, but not locked out.
- Keep the hips square and pull the abdominals in to avoid hollowing the lower back.
- Keep the spine long and the chest lifted.
- Lift the buttocks and push them backwards to increase the stretch at the back of the thigh.

## Progressions

- Start with a small range of motion by bending forwards only slightly.
- Progress to lifting the buttocks higher and increasing the forward bend, with the knee fully extended.
- Take a larger step forwards to increase the range of motion.

## Ex 2 | Front of thigh stretch

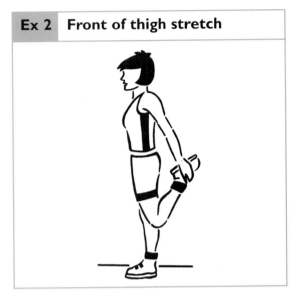

### Purpose

This exercise lengthens and stretches the quadriceps muscles at the front of the thigh. If the hips are tilted forwards, it will also stretch the hip flexor muscles (the iliopsoas).

### Starting position and instructions

Balance on one leg. Raise the heel of the opposite leg towards the buttock cheek. Use the hand to hold the leg and increase the range of motion. Hold still.

### Teaching points

- Use a wall or partner to assist balance.
- Keep the supporting knee joint unlocked.
- Only lift the leg to a point where a mild tension is felt at the front of the thigh; do not overflex (bend) the knee.
- Keep the hips facing forwards and avoid hollowing of the lower back by tightening the abdominal muscles.
- Lift the heel towards the centre of the buttock cheeks; avoid taking the heel to the outside of the buttocks as this may stress the ligaments on the inside of the knee.
- Tilt the hips slightly forwards.
- Keep both knees in line with each other.

### Progressions

- Start with a small range of motion by only raising the heel slightly. A towel can be used around the ankle to hold on to if desired.
- Keep the knee of the stretching leg slightly in front of the other knee to decrease the stretch.
- Progressively lift and move the heel closer to the buttocks to achieve a greater range of motion.
- Tilt the hips forwards to increase the stretch slightly.
- Take the knee of the stretching leg slightly back so that it is positioned to the side but slightly behind the other knee to increase the stretch.
- Bend and straighten the knee of the supporting leg while performing the stretch to add variety and motor skills.

## Ex 3 | Calf stretch

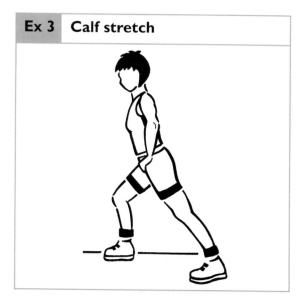

### Purpose

This exercise lengthens and stretches the gastrocnemius and soleus muscles at the back of the lower leg.

### Starting position and instructions

Start with the feet hip width apart. Step the left leg backwards as far as possible while keeping the heel of the left foot on the floor, and bend the right (front) knee.

### Teaching points

- Place the hands on a wall or hold a partner to assist balance.
- Keep the front knee bent but do not let the knee roll inwards.
- Keep the heel of the back foot facing forwards.
- Keep the hips facing forwards and avoid hollowing of the lower back by tucking in the buttock muscles.
- Keep the body upright, ensuring the hips do not bend forwards.
- Keep the chest lifted and the abdominals pulled in.

### Progressions

- For a smaller range of motion, only step the leg a small distance backwards.
- Combine with upper body stretches for variety, if motor skills allow.
- Lean into a wall while performing the stretch to increase the range of motion. Ensure correct alignment is maintained.

| Ex 4 | Inner thigh stretch |
|------|---------------------|

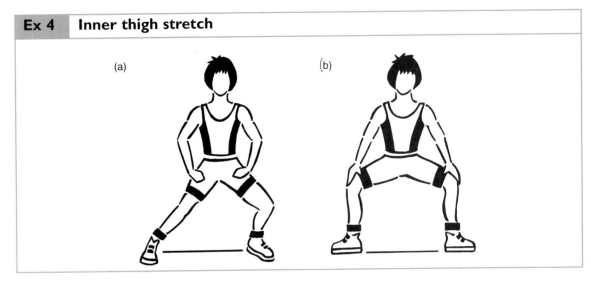

(a)　　(b)

## Purpose

This exercise lengthens and stretches the adductor muscles on the inside of the thigh.

## Starting position and instructions

Stand with the legs a shoulder width and a half apart, feet facing forwards or to the side, depending on which is more comfortable. A 45° angle is ideal. If the feet face forwards, take care not to place stress on the side of the ankle. Bend the left knee, taking the body weight towards the left. Keep the right knee straight but not locked (*see* figure a).

## Teaching points

- Use a wall to assist balance.
- Keep the knee joint of the weight-bearing leg unlocked, and the knee over the ankle and in line with the toes.
- Step the legs further apart to increase the stretch of the inner thigh and groin.
- Keep the hips facing forwards and avoid hollowing of the lower back by tucking in the buttock muscles.
- Position the foot of the stretching leg in a comfortable position, ideally keeping the knee in line with the toes.

## Progressions

- Start with a small range of motion with the legs only a small distance apart.
- Progress by stepping the legs further apart, but only to a point where correct alignment of the knees can be maintained.
- Tilt the pelvis sideways towards the weight-bearing knee to increase the stretch slightly.
- Combine with upper body stretches to add variety for individuals with greater motor skills.
- Stretch both legs together by squatting with the knees turned out, using the arms to press the knees out to the side (*see* figure b).

## Ex 5 Side stretch

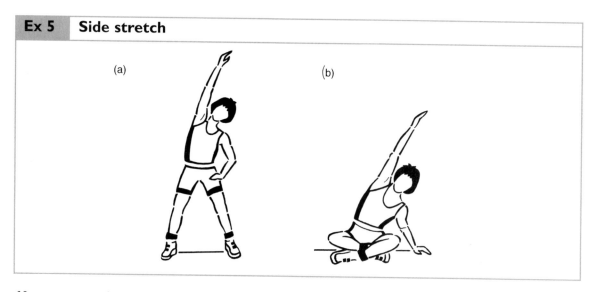

(a)　　　　　　　　　　(b)

*Note*: it is not advisable to perform this stretch with both arms out to the side. First, this palces a lot of unnecessary weight on the spine. Second, the muscles may not be able to relax and, therefore, may not stretch effectively.

### Purpose

This exercise lengthens and stretches the muscles at the sides of the trunk and the sides of the back (the obliques and latissimus dorsi).

### Starting position and instructions

Stand with the feet a shoulder width and a half apart, with the knees unlocked (*see* figure a). Place the left hand on the thigh to support the body weight. Lift the right arm up and bend over slightly to the left side. This can also be performed in a seated position (*see* figure b).

### Teaching points

- Keep both knee joints slightly bent.
- Emphasise the lifting of the body upwards as well as sideways to avoid leaning too far over to the side.
- Stretch only to a point where a mild tension is felt at the side of the trunk.
- Keep the hips facing forwards and avoid hollowing of the lower back by tucking in the buttock muscles.

- Keep the body weight equally placed between the two legs and avoid pushing the hip out to the side.
- When bending to the side, move the body in a straight line and do not lean forwards or backwards.
- Lift the rib cage up and create a gap between the pelvis and the ribs before bending to the side.

### Progressions

- Start by reaching up with the arm, not bending over to the side. Alternatively, keep both hands on the hips and bend over to the side which decreases the stretch slightly, and will take out any muscular work required of the shoulder to hold the arm up.
- Progress by reaching higher with the arm and bending over slightly further to achieve a greater range of motion. Ensure the correct alignment of the spine is maintained.

## Ex 6   Back of the upper arm stretch

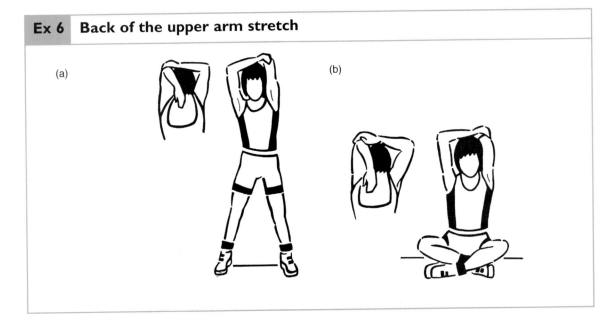

(a)   (b)

### Purpose

This exercise lengthens and stretches the triceps muscle at the back of the upper arm.

### Starting position and instructions

Stand with the feet hip width apart. Take one hand over the shoulder and place it in the centre of the back. Use the other arm to ease the arm further back by moving the elbow (*see* figure a). Hold still. This can also be performed in a seated position (*see* figure b).

### Teaching points

- Keep the knee joints slightly bent.
- Keep the hips facing forwards and avoid hollowing of the lower back by tucking in the buttock muscles and tightening the abdominal muscles.
- Stretch only to a point where a mild tension is felt at the back of the upper arm.

### Progressions

- For individuals with less flexibility, start with the hand on the shoulder and use the opposite hand to raise the arm up slightly and through a smaller range of motion.
- Progress by placing the palm of the hand in the centre of the back, using the other arm to ease the arm further back and downwards into the position.
- Progress further by taking the other arm behind the back into a half-nelson position and attempting to reach the fingers of the stretching arm. This will stretch the deltoid muscles at the front of the shoulder of the arm in the half-nelson position.
- Perform with a lower body stretch of the calves or adductors for variety, and if motor skills allow.

## Ex 7 Chest stretch

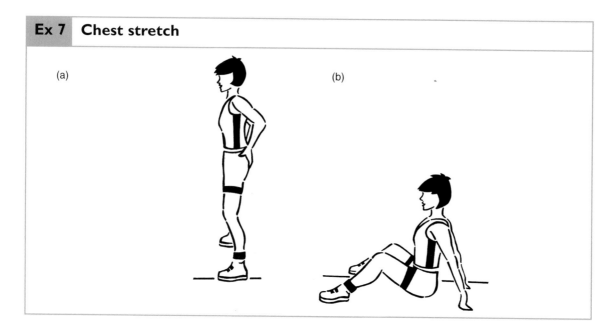

(a)                    (b)

### Purpose

This exercise lengthens and stretches the muscles of the chest (the pectorals).

### Starting position and instructions

Stand with the feet hip width apart. Take the hands backwards until a mild tension is felt at the front of the chest. The hands can be placed on the buttocks or clasped together behind the back, depending on which is most comfortable (*see* figure a). This can be performed in a seated position with the hands placed on the floor behind the back (*see* figure b).

### Teaching points

- Keep the knees unlocked.
- Keep the elbows slightly bent.
- Squeeze the shoulder blades together and lift the chest to increase the stretch.
- Keep the hips facing forwards and avoid hollowing of the lower back by tucking in the buttock muscles and tightening the abdominal muscles.

### Progressions

- Start with a small range of motion.
- Move the arms progressively through a greater range of motion by linking the fingers behind the back and lifting the arms up slightly.
- Taking the arms further back, allowing the hands to touch the buttocks, and squeezing the shoulder blades together will also increase the stretch for the pectorals.
- Perform with a lower body stretch of the calves or adductors to add variety, if motor skills allow.

## Ex 8 Middle back stretch

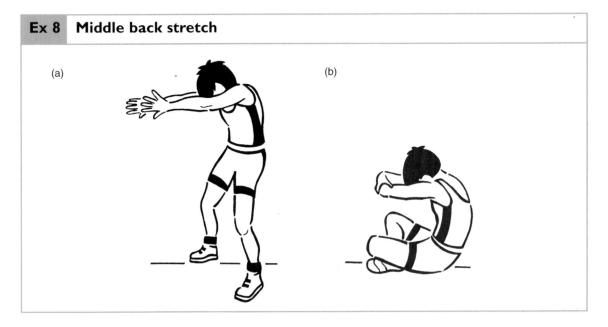

(a)

(b)

### Purpose

This exercise stretches the muscle in the middle of the back (the trapezius).

### Starting position and instructions

Stand with the feet a shoulder width and a half apart. Take both arms forwards in front of the body, just below shoulder height. Round the shoulders slightly to feel a mild tension in the middle of the upper back (*see* figure a). This can be performed in a seated position, with the arms crossed in front of the body and hands gripping the elbows (*see* figure b).

### Teaching points

- Keep the knees unlocked.
- Keep the elbows slightly bent.
- Keep the hips facing forwards and avoid hollowing of the lower back by tucking in the buttock muscles and tightening the abdominal muscles.
- Round the shoulders slightly without leaning forwards at the hips.

### Progressions

- Start with a small range of motion by not rounding the shoulders very far.
- Move the arms progressively through a greater range of motion by rounding the shoulders further.
- Wrapping the arms around the body at the front with the hands touching the back (hugging yourself) will increase the stretch even further.
- Perform with a lower body stretch of the calves or adductors to add variety, if motor skills allow.

# DESIGNING A COOL-DOWN

## Why do we need to cool down?

We need to cool down after the main workout to return all the bodily systems to their pre-exercise state. It is, therefore, essential that appropriate time is set aside for cooling down after the main workout. At the end of the cool-down we should feel refreshed, rejuvenated, and motivated to return to future sessions, so it is important that the appropriate and correct exercises are selected. This chapter discusses what should happen to the body during this concluding component of the session (the short-term physiological responses). It also outlines how to design a safe and effective cool-down.

## What types of exercises should the cool-down contain?

The cool-down needs to include exercises that return the body to its pre-exercise state by achieving the desired effects outlined in table 6.1.

## What types of exercises are appropriate to lower the pulse and cool down?

Exercises that progressively reduce the intensity of the activities used throughout the main workout will effectively lower the heart rate, breathing rate and the body temperature. This can be achieved easily by starting the component with larger movements that continue the intensity of the main workout, then gradually reducing the intensity of each

| Table 6.1 | The desired effects of the cool-down on the body |
| --- | --- |

The cool-down should be characterised by the following.

- It should gradually lower and return the heart rate to a pre-exercise level. This reduces the stress on the heart muscle. It also promotes the return of venous blood to the heart, lowering the risk of blood pooling. This can be achieved by **pulse-lowering/cooling-down** exercises.
- It should lengthen the muscles back to their normal state. This will maintain the flexibility and range of motion of the muscles and joints. This can be achieved by static **maintenance stretches**.
- It should increase the length of the muscles. This will increase the flexibility and range of motion of the joints and muscles. This can be achieved by static **developmental stretches**.
- It should relax the body and mind. This will help to reduce stress and promote a feeling of serenity. This can be achieved by specific **relaxation** techniques.
- It should revitalise the body and mind. This will leave the body feeling rejuvenated and ready to return to normal activities. This can be achieved by gentle **re-mobilising** exercises.

exercise. Reducing the speed of the exercises, performing them with shallower bends, travelling less and moving through a smaller range of motion will lower the intensity of each movement. Care should be taken not to reduce the intensity too quickly as this would give the heart little time to adapt and can be very stressful and potentially dangerous. It is always advisable to slow down gradually.

## How will pulse-lowering and cooling-down exercises alter for different groups?

Although less fit and specialist groups will be working at a relatively low intensity in the main workout, they will need to spend slightly longer cooling down because it generally takes their bodies longer to recover from the demands of the workout. The intensity at which the cool-down starts for a less fit group will therefore need to be lower, and more time should be spent on decreasing the intensity.

Fitter groups will be working at a higher intensity in the main workout, but despite this they can still cool down, and at a more rapid pace because their body systems are more efficient. The intensity of the cool-down for a fitter group can therefore start at a much higher level and decrease more quickly.

## What types of exercises are appropriate to stretch the muscles?

Exercises that allow the muscles to relax and lengthen are appropriate. This can be achieved by performing a combination of the static or moving stretches that are used for the preparatory (warm-up) stretch; these are outlined in chapter 5. Both types of stretches will fulfil the main requirement of the post-workout stretch, which is to lengthen the muscles after work and maintain their range of motion. Static stretches are more appropriate to enhance the development of a relaxed state.

To improve flexibility, developmental stretches would need to be included in the cool-down. Developmental stretches are those where the muscle is stretched to a point at which a mild tension is experienced and then held still. When the tension eases, the muscle can then be lengthened further by moving to a greater range of motion. This process can be repeated a few times, moving even further into the stretch every time the tension eases. Once a comfortable but extended range of motion is achieved, the stretch should be held for as long as is comfortable. This will help develop a greater range of motion. The positions used for developmental stretches should be as comfortable and relaxed as possible. Seated or lying positions are often the most appropriate since they reduce the amount of muscle work required to hold the body in a specific position.

Floor-based post-workout stretches are illustrated with step-by-step instructions later in this chapter (*see* pages 72–80). The preparatory stretches illustrated in chapter 5 (*see* pages 59–66) may also be used for post-workout stretches. These include upper and lower body stretches in standing positions.

## Which muscles need to be stretched?

All muscles will need to be stretched and lengthened after work, so stretches should be included for all the muscles used in the main workout. The stretch positions illustrated at the end of this chapter are the most appropriate for post-workout stretching. The floor-based positions that are illustrated are generally more comfortable and relaxing than the standing stretch positions illustrated at the end of chapter 5. However, if the room is cooler, or if the stretches are just intended to maintain flexibility, then standing stretches are also appropriate.

If the main workout is very intense, it can be beneficial to include extra stretches for the muscles that have worked the hardest throughout. However, the level of activity and number of stretches included will also depend on the temperature of the room. If the room is cooler, it is advisable to keep the number of stretches to a minimum, but to ensure that all the muscles worked have been stretched. It may be more effective to stretch some muscles after the cardio-vascular workout, and some muscles after the muscular strength and endurance component, rather than leaving the stretching of all the muscles to the end of the session. This will prevent the body cooling down too quickly and getting cold. If the body does get too cold the muscles will not be stretching effectively.

## What types of exercises are appropriate to relax the body and mind?

Exercises that do not require excessive muscular work and allow the mind to relax are most effective. There are various relaxation techniques that can be used. These include the tense and release method, the extend and release method, and the visualisation method. Each method can be just as effective so it is advisable to utilise a variety of the techniques.

### Tense and release

This can be achieved by tensing the muscles in a specific body area, holding for a short duration, and then releasing the tension and allowing the area to relax. For example, flexing the foot so the toes point towards the knee will tense the muscle at the front of the shin (tibialis anterior) and relax the muscles of the calf (gastrocnemius and soleus). Working through each part of the body is preferable to tensing the whole body. In some instances the latter can make you feel more tense.

### Extend and release

This can be achieved by extending the muscles in a specific body area, holding the position for a short time, and then relaxing the position. For example, in a comfortable position, press the feet away from the head, hold the position then release the position.

### Visualisation

This can be achieved by mentally visualising a situation or place where you always feel relaxed. No specific scenario is recommended because each individual will react differently to different environments.

Ultimately, the appropriateness of specific relaxation techniques will depend upon the temperature of the room and the requirements of the group. In a cold room it is unlikely participants will be able to relax; they will be more concerned about keeping warm. In addition, some participants will not like performing these activities so the teacher should explain the benefits which can be achieved if the body is able to relax. It is worthwhile including a short relaxation component in all etm sessions just to give the mind and body time to do absolutely nothing and to just lie still.

## What types of exercises are appropriate to re-mobilise the body?

At the end of the session participants should leave feeling refreshed, sufficiently warm, and motivated to return to another session. Therefore, low-intensity versions of the mobility exercises illustrated in chapter 5 can be appropriate to re-mobilise the body. It can also be quite effective to prepare a fun sequence to finish the session, but a themed re-mobiliser may not appeal to all participants. Whatever approach is used, it is advisable to make the movements slightly less energetic at this stage of the session. The aim is not to prepare the body for a workout but to prepare it for returning to daily life.

The time spent re-mobilising the body will depend on the duration of the relaxation and post-workout stretch components. If a long time has been dedicated to these components, then an equal amount of time will be needed to re-mobilise the body.

## What factors will affect the overall timing and intensity of the cool-down?

- Temperature.
- Intensity of the main workout.
- Age and ability of the participants.

### Temperature

The body will cool down much more quickly when the room or weather is cold, so it is wise to use only maintenance stretches and to leave out any relaxation exercises in cold temperatures. Alternatively, if participants have tracksuits with them they can put them on before moving into the stretch and relaxation components. This may disrupt the flow of the class so careful planning is needed to maintain a relaxed atmosphere.

### Intensity of the main workout

For sessions containing a cardio-vascular train-ing component, the duration spent lowering intensity after the main component will vary: if the intensity of the main workout is relatively high, then a longer period of time will need to be spent lowering the intensity; if the intensity is low, then the duration can generally be shorter.

However, the duration will also depend on the fitness level of the participants (see opposite). Once the heart rate is lowered, the muscles that are no longer going to be worked can be stretched. It may also be advisable to include additional stretches for muscles that have received a lot of work in the main workout.

If the preceding workout consists mainly of muscular strength and endurance exercises, for example a body conditioning or sculpt class, then the cool-down will not need to start at such a high intensity and less time will be needed to lower the intensity. Some less intense muscular strength and endurance activities may, in fact, have a cooling effect on the body, so rather than cooling down it may be necessary to re-warm the body prior to post-exercise stretching.

Sessions combining cardio-vascular and muscular strength and endurance training will normally be structured so that the main pulse-lowering exercises follow the cardio-vascular workout. The muscular strength and endurance work will follow these exercises and will generally be floor-based. Therefore, stretching activities can directly follow this component provided the body is still sufficiently warm.

### The age and ability of participants

Less fit and specialist groups will need to spend slightly longer cooling down. They will need to spend longer lowering the intensity after cardio-vascular training to allow for effective recovery. They will also need longer to get into and out of stretch positions and will often need more careful coaching on how to get into and out of these positions.

## How should the cool-down be structured for an etm session?

The cool-down should be structured in four stages:

1 cooling-down/pulse-lowering exercises
2 post-workout stretches – maintenance and developmental
3 relaxation
4 re-mobilise.

### Summary of the guidelines for planning the cool-down

- Plan for pulse-lowering exercises to follow any cardio-vascular training. Start with high-intensity exercises and gradually build down the range of motion and intensity of the movements. This can be achieved by progressively decreasing the amount of jumping, bending, and travelling movements and moving at a progressively slower pace.
- Muscular strength and endurance-based classes generally will not need to include pulse-lowering exercises. However, a short time may need to be spent lowering the heart rate following any intense lower body work, i.e. Squats, Dead Lifts and Lunges.
- Maintenance stretches should be included for all the muscles worked in the main workout.
- Developmental stretches should be included for muscle groups which lack a full range of motion. Comfortable and supportive positions should be used when developing a stretch and the muscle must be sufficiently warm.
- Only include specific relaxation exercises if the room temperature is warm.
- For re-mobilising use gentle exercises that will enliven the body and mind and finish the session on a positive note.
- In a traditional class structure the muscular strength and endurance training will generally come between the pulse-lowering exercises which follow cardio-vascular training, and the post-workout stretch component.

# POST-WORKOUT STRETCHES

The stretch positions illustrated in this section are appropriate for preparatory as well as post-workout stretching. However, in the warm-up the room temperature and possible interruptions to class flow if using floor-based stretches should be considered so that the benefits of the warm-up are not lost. Specific stretches for the upper body are illustrated in both a standing and seated position in chapter 5.

| Ex 1 | Back of thigh stretch (lying) |
|---|---|

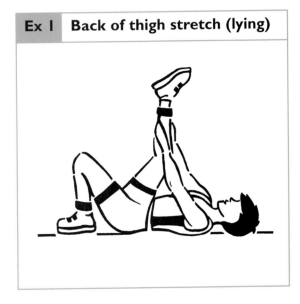

## Purpose

This exercise lengthens and stretches the hamstring muscles at the back of the thigh, and also the buttock muscles (the gluteals).

## Starting position and instructions

Lie on the back with the knees bent and the feet firmly on the floor. Raise one leg towards the chest and hold it at the back of the thigh or calf, wherever is most comfortable. Use the hand to support the leg and achieve a fuller range of motion. Hold still.

To develop the stretch, allow the tension to ease and then use the hands to guide the leg into a larger range of motion.

## Teaching points

- Keep the lower back on the floor.
- Only lift the leg to a point where a mild tension is felt at the back of the thigh.
- Aim to fully extend the knee of the stretching leg.
- Keep the head and shoulders supported on the floor.
- Keep the knee joint of the other leg bent.

## Progressions

- Start with a small range of motion by not lifting the leg very high. Use a towel if necessary to hold around the leg.
- Keep the knee slightly bent if fully extending the knee is uncomfortable.
- Progress by lifting the leg closer to the chest.

## Ex 2 | Front of thigh stretch (lying)

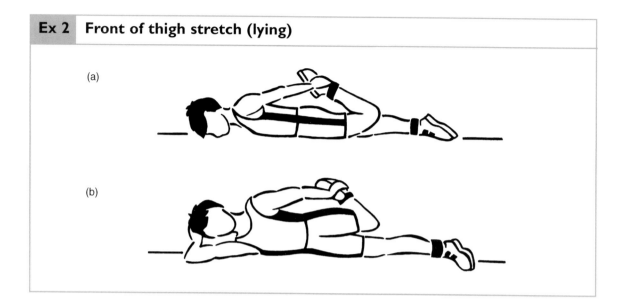

(a)

(b)

## Purpose

This exercise lengthens and stretches the quadriceps muscles at the front of the thigh. If the hips are tilted forwards, it will also stretch the hip flexor muscles (the iliopsoas).

## Starting position and instructions

Lie either (a) on the tummy or (b) on one side. Raise the heel of one leg (the top leg in the case of a side lying position) towards the centre of the buttock cheek. Use the hand to hold the leg and achieve a fuller range of motion. Hold still. To develop the stretch, hold until the tension eases and then take the knee further back and press the hips forwards.

## Teaching points

- Only lift the leg to a point where a mild tension is felt at the front of the thigh; do not overflex (bend) the knee.
- Keep the back straight and abdominal muscles pulled in.
- Keep the hips facing forwards and avoid hollowing of the lower back.

- Lift the heel towards the centre of the buttock cheeks; avoid taking the heel to the outside of the buttocks as this may stress the ligaments on the inside of the knee.
- Tilt the hips slightly forwards.
- Aim to keep both knees in line with each other.

## Progressions

- It may be easier for less flexible participants to lie on their side. This allows the knee to be positioned slightly in front of the body and the range of motion to be smaller.
- A towel can be used to hold the ankle and decrease the range of motion.
- Progressively lift the heel towards the buttocks to achieve a greater range of motion.
- Tilt the hips forwards to increase the stretch slightly.
- Take the knee of the stretching leg slightly back, so that it is positioned to the side but slightly behind the other knee, to increase the stretch.

## Ex 3 Calf stretch

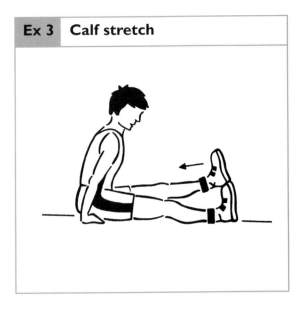

## Purpose

This exercise lengthens and stretches the gastrocnemius and soleus muscles at the back of the lower leg.

## Starting position and instructions

Sit up straight with the legs in front of the body. If it is more comfortable to lean slightly backwards the arms should be placed on the floor behind the body to support the body weight. Place the heel of one foot over the toe of the other foot and use the top leg to ease the toes towards the body, stretching the calf muscle.

## Teaching points

- Keep the knee joints of both legs unlocked.
- Only move to a point where a mild tension is felt in the calf.
- Keep the hips facing forwards and avoid hollowing of the lower back by tightening the abdominal muscles.
- Keep the shoulders relaxed and down.

## Progressions

- Move through a small range of motion by easing the toes only a small distance towards the body.
- Ease the toes closer to the body to achieve a greater range of motion.
- Use the hands to reach forwards and ease the foot towards the body. *Note*: only participants who have flexible hamstrings will be able to do this.
- As a variation, perform the same stretch lying on the back.

## Ex 4  Inner thigh stretch (seated)

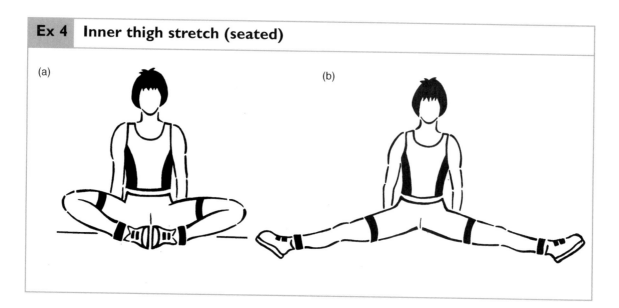

(a)                                    (b)

## Purpose

This exercise lengthens and stretches the adductor muscles on the inside of the thigh.

## Starting position and instructions

Sit on the floor with either (a) the soles of the feet together, or (b) with the legs straddled out wide. The hands can be placed on the floor behind the back to help maintain an upright position of the spine. Flexible participants who are able to keep their spine upright can keep the hands on the floor in front of the body (straddle), or on the knees (soles of feet together).

## Teaching points

- Keep the back straight and the chest lifted.
- Visualise the vertebrae as bricks and the vertebrae discs as marshmallows to maintain an upright spine.
- Move the legs to a point where a mild tension is felt inside of the thigh and groin.
- Keep the hips facing forwards and avoid hollowing of the lower back.
- Breathe.

## Progressions

- Start with a small range of motion in the straddle position by not taking the legs out very far. Progress by taking the legs wider apart.
- Start with a small range of motion in the soles of feet together position by keeping the feet further away from the body and easing the knees only a small distance towards the floor. Progress by bringing the feet closer to the body and easing the knees further down towards the floor.
- Both positions can be performed lying on the back. Note: if lying on the back with the legs straddled and raised in the air, ensure that the legs stay in line with the belly button and support the weight of the legs by holding the outside of the knees with the hands. This will allow the muscles to relax more easily.
- Another lying alternative is to bring the knees towards the arm pits with the soles of the feet together or slightly apart.

## Ex 5    Back of thigh stretch (seated)

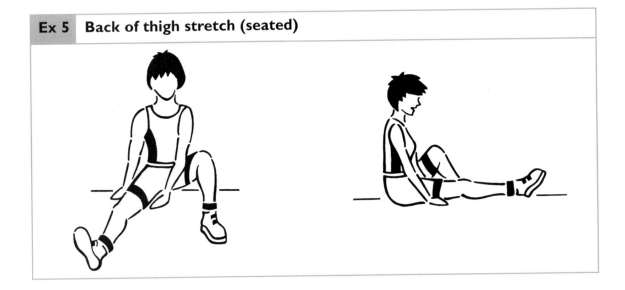

### Purpose

This exercise lengthens and stretches the muscles at the back of the thigh (the hamstrings).

### Starting position and instructions

Sit upright with one leg out straight in front of the body and the other leg out to the side. Bend forwards from the hips, feeling a stretch in the back of the thigh. The hands can be kept behind the back to keep the spine supported for less flexible participants, otherwise place them either side of the outstretched leg.

### Teaching points

- Keep the knee of the stretching leg slightly bent.
- Emphasise lifting the body upwards as well as forwards, and stretch to a point where a mild tension is felt at the back of the thigh.

- Keep the chest lifted and the abdominal muscles pulled in.
- Ensure the other leg is in a comfortable position. Avoid the hurdle position (where the foot of the bent leg is placed next to the buttock) as this may place stress on the ligaments at the inside of the knee joint.

### Progressions

- Start by only bending slightly forwards.
- Progress by gradually bending further to achieve a greater range of motion.
- Push the buttocks backwards to increase the stretch.
- Both legs can be stretched at the same time if participants are flexible enough. However, it should be noted that the range of motion will be limited to the range achievable by the least flexible muscle.

## Ex 6 | Hip flexor stretch

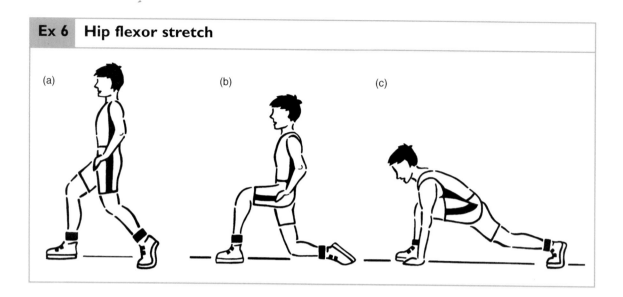

(a)        (b)        (c)

### Purpose

This exercise lengthens and stretches the iliopsoas muscle, which runs through to the front of the femur (thigh bone) from the pelvis and the lumbar spine.

### Starting position and instructions

(a) Stand with the feet hip width apart. Step back with the left leg, bend both knees and lift the left heel off the floor. (b) Kneel on the floor. Step one leg forwards into a lunge position with the foot flat on the floor. Keep the other knee on the floor and press the hips forwards to feel a stretch through the hip. The hands can rest on the hips, or on the floor to assist balance. Keep the chest lifted.

### Teaching points

- Keep the back straight.
- Keep the hips facing forwards.
- Stretch only to a point where a mild tension is felt.
- Keep the knee of the front leg in line with the ankle.
- Ensure the knee does not overshoot the toe.

### Progressions

- Less flexible participants can perform this stretch standing up, with one leg back slightly and the hips tilted forwards. This can be progressed by gradually taking the leg further back.
- The rear knee can be lifted from the floor if this is more comfortable (*see* figure c). However, this tends to make the stretch position more active. This position can be progressed by first taking the legs a small distance apart and then gradually taking the legs to a further, but comfortable, distance apart.
- Tilt the pelvis forwards while performing the stretch to increase the range of motion slightly.

| Ex 7 | Outside of hip and thigh stretch |
|---|---|

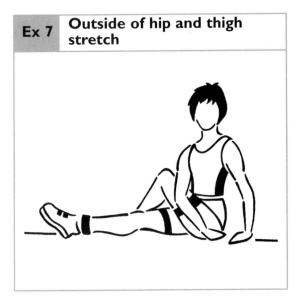

## Purpose

This exercise lengthens and stretches the muscles at the side of the hip and thigh (the abductors). It may also provide some stretch for the muscles at the sides of the back, and in the lower back (erector spinae).

## Starting position and instructions

Sit upright with both legs out in front of the body. Bend the left knee and cross it over the right leg, placing the left foot on the floor by the side of the right knee. Lift the chest up and twist the body towards the left, placing the right elbow against the left knee to ease the stretch further.

## Teaching points

- Keep the spine upright.
- Keep the hips facing forwards and avoid hollowing of the lower back.
- Twist the body from the trunk, keeping the buttocks firmly placed on the floor.
- Rotate around only as far as is comfortable.

## Progressions

- Start with a small range of motion by not twisting the body very far.
- Move progressively to a greater range of motion by twisting further and using the arm to ease the leg further away from the direction in which the body is turning.

## Ex 8 | Back stretch

(a)                    (b)

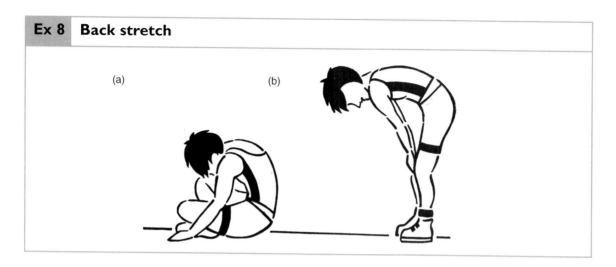

## Purpose

This exercise lengthens and stretches the muscles of the back (the erector spinae).

## Starting position and instructions

Sit upright with the legs crossed in front of the body. Bend the body forwards and curl the spine, lengthening the neck and whole of the spine (*see* figure (a). This exercise can also be performed in a standing position by leaning forwards, placing the hands on the knees and rounding the back and neck (*see* figure (b).

## Teaching points

• Keep the spine curled and relaxed.
• Keep the buttock muscles firmly on the floor.
• Keep the hands on the floor to support the weight of the body.
• Only stretch to a point where a mild tension is felt.

## Progressions

• Start with a small range of motion, by bending forwards only slightly.
• Move progressively to a greater range of motion by bending further forwards.
• Participants who can bend forwards comfortably through a large range of motion can place their hands at the back of the head to increase the stretch in this area.
• Move the legs further from the body if sitting cross-legged is not comfortable.

## Ex 9 Rectus abdominus stretch

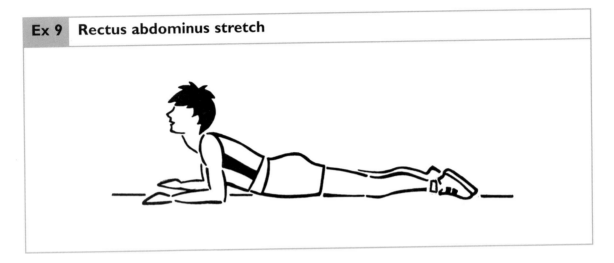

### Purpose

To stretch the muscles at the front of the tummy (rectus abdominus)

### Instructions

Lie on tummy (prone lying)
Elbows and forearms on floor.
Hands level with shoulders.
Lengthen the body forward and raise onto the elbows to stretch the abdominals.
Hold and return to start position.

### Teaching points

- Relax the legs.
- Keep the shoulders lengthened.
- Look forward slightly.
- Care not to hyperextend (excessively arch) the spine too much
- Lift only to a position that is comfortable

### Alternative

- Lie on back and reach arms overhead along floor, allowing back to arch slightly
- Lift the elbows off the floor to increase the stretch. Extend the elbow to simulate the cobra pose (yoga). However, this may cause the spine to hyperextend too much for certain individuals.

# APPROACHES TO EXERCISE
## TO MUSIC

# PART THREE

# DESIGNING A CARDIO-VASCULAR TRAINING PROGRAMME

7

## How should a cardio-vascular training session be structured?

There is a variety of different approaches to cardio-vascular training: aerobics, step, hi-lo, cardio-funk are just a few of the alternatives adopted by teachers. The structure of these specific sessions should be the same regardless of the approach adopted: a thorough warm-up and stretch should precede the main workout, and a comprehensive cool-down and post-work-out should conclude the session. An appropriate session structure is outlined in table 7.1.

The exercises selected, however, will need to be adapted to suit each approach. To improve the fitness of the heart, lungs and circulatory system, the exercises selected for the main workout need to be performed at a higher level of intensity and should create a feeling of mild breathlessness.

This chapter discusses how to structure each specific component to achieve a safe and effective cardio-vascular training session. It also illustrates a variety of exercises that can be performed in a traditional hi-lo aerobic session. A list of progressions is included for each exercise, which allows for the choreography to be altered. Specific exercises and guidelines for structuring a step training programme are illustrated in chapter 8.

## What types of exercises are appropriate to re-warm the body and increase the intensity for cardio-vascular training?

The re-warmer (build-up aerobics) should commence with less intense versions of the exercises to be performed in the main component. The intensity of each exercise will then need to be built up progressively to the desired level. This can be achieved by starting with relatively small movements and gradually increasing the size of the movement. Gradually moving the centre of gravity in more of an upwards (jumping), downwards (bending the knees) or travelling (walking, running) direction are effective methods of increasing intensity to improve cardio-vascular fitness. Increasing the speed of the movement sequences by using a slightly faster music tempo, using additional muscle groups (combining arm lines with leg work), and lengthening levers (straight leg kicks instead of knee raises) are also effective ways of increasing the intensity of specific exercises.

| Table 7.1 | The structure of a session to train cardio-vascular fitness |
|---|---|
| Warm-up | • Mobility and pulse-raising exercises.<br>• Preparatory stretches. |
| Main workout (1):<br>cardio-vascular training (essential) | • Re-warmer (build-up aerobics) to raise the intensity (elevate heart rate into training zone).<br>• Maintenance of intensity (maintain heart rate within the recommended training zone).<br>• Pulse-lowering exercises to lower intensity (lower the heart rate out of the training zone) and promote venous return. |
| Main workout (2): muscular<br>strength and endurance training (optional) | • Specific toning exercises for muscle groups not targeted in main session. This will generally require the upper body muscles (back, arms, chest and abdominals) to be prioritised to achieve muscle balance in the session. |
| Cool-down | • Post-workout stretches (maintenance and developmental).<br>• Relaxation (optional).<br>• Re-mobilise. |

*Note*: If muscular strength and endurance exercises are included, the session will follow the traditional ETM session format and will include training all the components of fitness.

## What factors will affect the rate at which the intensity can be increased?

The rate at which the intensity can be increased will depend primarily on the fitness of the participants. Less fit and specialist groups will generally need slightly longer to increase intensity than a fitter group because their heart and circulatory systems are unable to cope with intense activities. It is advisable for less fit and specialist groups to start off at a low intensity and build up to a moderate intensity. This will enable them to utilise the aerobic energy system and to work out for longer and more comfortably.

A fitter group will have a more effective heart and circulatory system. Their heart muscle will be stronger and will be able to pump and circulate the blood more effectively to the muscles. The muscles will be more able to utilise the oxygen being supplied and will be physiologically equipped to remove waste products more effectively. A fitter group will therefore be able to start at a higher level of intensity and progress more quickly to work at a harder pace and for a longer duration through the main cardio-vascular component.

The progression of this component will also depend on the intensity maintained throughout the preparatory stretch component. If the body is kept fairly active, and the intensity is maintained at a reasonable level throughout that component, it is unlikely that much time will need to be spent re-warming. The intensity can therefore be raised to a higher level at a slightly faster pace by performing frequent pulse-raising moves in between static stretching exercises. However, it should be noted that the skill level and experience of participants will affect whether they are able to exercise safely and effectively in this way, so discretion should be used. It may be necessary for a less skilled group to have less frequent pulse-raising exercises to ensure they concentrate sufficiently on achieving a safe and effective stretch. In this instance, the intensity of the re-warmer will perhaps need to be slightly lower to ensure the intensity is able to build up progressively and effectively.

## What types of exercises are appropriate to maintain the intensity?

Exercises that require the use of the large muscle groups and maintain a constant intensity and a mild state of breathlessness are appropriate. Oxygen consumption is generally higher during travelling, jumping and bending movements because the large leg muscles are responsible for shifting the centre of gravity and moving the weight of the body in each direction. The deeper one bends, the higher one jumps and the further one travels, the greater will be the intensity. This will require the cardio-vascular system to respond by delivering more oxygen to the muscles. An appropriate range of exercises are illustrated at the end of this chapter. Each exercise can be travelled or jumped to further increase intensity so they are all very effective for maintaining the heart rate in the training zone. In addition, some of the pulse-raising exercises illustrated in

chapter 5, such as travelling Side Squats and Grapevines, can be effective if they are performed at a high intensity.

Movements of the upper body demand lower volumes of oxygen than movements of the lower body because the muscles involved (deltoids etc.) are smaller and the weight and leverage they are moving (the arms) are lighter. Upper body movements, therefore, place less demands on the cardio-vascular system. Often the heart rate will increase slightly when the arms are used, especially if they are moved above the head, however this response is due to the heart needing to pump blood upwards against the force of gravity, rather than demanding the supply of a larger volume of oxygen, the latter being the primary intention of effective cardio-vascular training.

Upper body movements (arm lines) are illustrated with instructions at the end of this chapter. These can be used in conjunction with the cardio-vascular exercises for the lower body that are also illustrated.

While movements of the legs are most effective to bring about the desired training effect, too much repetition of the same movement may cause unnecessary stress on the joints. Jumping movements (high impact), in particular, place a lot of stress on the weight-bearing joints because the velocity at which the body lands will cause impact forces that will be absorbed by the body. Cushioning each jumping movement by softening the knees and allowing the heels to go down will dissipate these forces to some extent. However, the weight of the individual and the strength of their muscles will also affect whether they can perform jumping movements safely. A heavier person with relatively weak muscles will have more weight being borne by the joints, and if their muscles are not sufficiently strong to maintain correct alignment, jumping activities may cause injury. Individuals with strong muscles who are able to maintain correct joint alignment, and individuals with a lighter body weight, are less at risk when performing high-impact jumping exercises.

Bending movements are low impact by nature but can be equally stressful on the joints. Repetitive bending of the joints in the same direction, for example lots of squatting and lunging movements, may cause repetitive strain. As the muscles that support the joint become fatigued, correct joint alignment may be lost, potentially causing further stress to the tissues (ligaments and tendons) around this area. Ideally, the movements and the muscle work should be varied to avoid fatigue and maintain the safety and effectiveness of the session.

Travelling movements often involve more muscles, but even though more muscles share the stress, some will still be working harder than others. Too much repetition of the same joint actions in the same direction, for example continuous lateral (sideways) squatting, may place unnecessary stress on the ligaments inside and outside of the knee joint (medial and lateral ligaments). Continuous movement in the same direction and using the same muscles should therefore not be continued for long durations.

Ultimately, the less repetitious and more varied the movements throughout this component, the safer will be the workout. However, one must consider that too many changes of movement may become confusing for participants with less effective motor skills. A balance needs to be achieved to maximise overall safety and effectiveness. Varying the directions of travelling movements and combining a mixture of jumping (high-impact) and squatting (low-impact) exercises throughout the session will generally bring about the desired training effect and maintain the safety of the workout.

## How will fitness levels affect the intensity maintained?

The intensity maintained and the duration for which it is maintained, will very much depend on the level of fitness of the participant. Less fit and specialist groups will need to work at a lower intensity and for a shorter duration than a fitter group. They should perform their higher intensity exercises at less frequent intervals throughout the component to allow them time to recover and to ensure they feel comfortable throughout the workout.

Participants in a fitter group will have more effective cardio-vascular systems so they should be able to work at a higher-intensity for a longer duration. Any high-intensity activities can be performed at more frequent intervals, and a comparatively longer time can be spent performing each activity; the duration of the whole component can also be slightly longer.

It is worth reiterating at this point that an activity that is easy for a fitter group may well be very intense for a less fit and specialist group. Therefore, careful consideration should be given to selecting the intensity when dealing with lower fitness levels. It is advisable to exclude the high-intensity exercises, such as those which require the body to move explosively (Power Jumps and Leaps), when dealing with these groups as they are very demanding and require a greater skill level. A range of progressions are detailed for all the exercises illustrated at the end of this chapter, and it may be appropriate to offer less fit groups modified versions of the more intense activities. As a general guideline, the intensity of most movements can be lowered by reducing the height of jumps, reducing the depth of bends, travelling less, using shorter levers, moving at a slower pace and generally exerting less energy.

## How will I know the intensity of the exercise?

There are various ways of monitoring the intensity of an exercise, and heart rate monitoring is one of them. Maintaining the heart or pulse rate somewhere between 55% and 90% of its maximum beats per minute is suggested as an appropriate training range. An individual's maximum heart rate can be estimated by subtracting their age from 220. For example, the maximal heart rate for a 30-year-old would be 190 beats per minute. This is outlined in table 7.2.

| Table 7.2 | Maximum heart rate and training zone for a 30-year-old |
|---|---|

220 – 30 (age) = 190 beats per minute (maximum heart rate)
10% of this maximum = 19 bpm (approx.)

To calculate the training zone, multiply 19 (10% of the maximal heart rate) by 5.5 (55%) and 9 (90%)

55% of this maximum = 104 bpm (approx.)
(Calculation: 10% of maximal heart rate × 5.5)
90% of this maximum = 171 bpm (approx.)
(Calculation: 10% of maximal heart rate × 9)

Therefore, the training zone for a 30-year-old would be between 104 and 171 bpm. That is, they should work between this range in the main workout to improve their cardio-vascular fitness.

However, accurate heart rate monitoring is not easy and it takes a lot of practice to obtain a reasonably accurate reading. Frequently, the heart rate is miscalculated by missing beats at the start and finish of the count, hearing and counting echo beats within the count and/or counting the movements of the legs instead of the heart rate. (Note: it is essential to keep the legs moving to avoid blood pooling – this will be discussed later in this chapter – and less experienced individuals can often count the movement of their legs by mistake.) Therefore, it may be more appropriate to use an alternative method of monitoring intensity. Two alternative methods for monitoring workout intensity are the talk test and the perceived rate of exertion.

## Talk test

Working to a level where one can breathe comfortably, rhythmically, and hold a conversation while exercising is suggested to indicate an appropriate intensity. A guideline for using the talk test is provided in table 7.3.

## Perceived rate of exertion (pre)

Borg (1982) researched and developed the ratio PRE category scale. This is outlined in table 7.4. The scale provides a range of intensity levels from 0 to 10. An easy-to-remember verbal expression is used to suggest how the intensity of an activity is perceived by the performer. When the activity is perceived to be 'strong' (a rating between 4 and 7 on the scale), Borg suggests it should correspond to an appropriate intensity for improving cardio-vascular fitness.

The accuracy of any of the aforementioned approaches is questionable and should only be used as a guideline on how hard a person is working. It is advisable to use a combination of the methods described for monitoring intensity and to be constantly vigilant for signs of overexertion, such as heavy breathing and excessive pallor or flushing of the skin.

| Table 7.3 | Using the talk test to monitor intensity | |
|---|---|---|
| Intensity level | Talk test response while performing an exercise | Action |
| Too high | If one or only a few words can be spoken | Lower the intensity immediately |
| Too low | If a number of sentences can be spoken too comfortably | Increase the intensity |
| Appropriate | If a mild breathlessness is apparent at the end of speaking a couple of sentences | Maintain this level of intensity |

| Table 7.4 | Using ratio perceived rate of exertion to monitor intensity | |
|---|---|---|
| Scale | Intensity | Verbal expression to describe the perceived intensity of activity |
| 0 | Nothing at all | |
| 0.5 | Extremely light | Just noticeable |
| 1 | Very light | |
| 2 | Light | Weak |
| 3 | Moderate | |
| 4 | Somewhat heavy | |
| 5 | Heavy | Strong |
| 6 | | |
| 7 | Very heavy | |
| 8 | | |
| 9 | | |
| 10 | Extremely heavy | Almost maximal |
| | Maximal | |

## When might it be necessary to stop exercising?

Exercise should be stopped, and it would be advisable to consult a doctor, if:

- normal co-ordination is lost while exercising
- dizziness occurs during exercise
- breathing difficulties are experienced
- tightness in the chest is experienced
- any other pain is experienced.

## What types of exercises are appropriate to lower the pulse and the intensity?

Exercises that progressively slow down the heart rate and breathing rate are appropriate, and this can be achieved by commencing with the exercises used in the previous component to maintain the intensity, progressively making the movements less intense. Reducing the number of jumping, travelling and deep bending movements, moving at a progressively slower pace, exerting less energy and utilising shorter levers (smaller kicks and arm movements) will all lower the intensity.

Progressively lowering the heart rate in this manner reduces the stress on the heart muscle and promotes the return of venous blood to the heart. This reduces the risk of blood pooling in the extremities which can occur if intense activities are stopped suddenly and the heart continues to pump out the same volume of blood, but there is no movement of the muscles of the lower body to assist the return of blood. It is, therefore, essential to maintain a certain amount of movement of the legs until the heart rate is sufficiently lowered out of the training zone.

## What factors will affect the rate at which the intensity can be lowered?

A less fit group will need to spend slightly longer lowering their heart rate effectively, even though they would not have been working at such a high intensity in the main workout. This allows their bodies sufficient time to recover and reduces the stress placed on the heart muscle. A fitter group should generally recover at a quicker rate. They should be able to cool down from a much higher intensity much quicker without placing stress on the heart. Their cardio-vascular systems will be better equipped to return venous blood to the heart.

## Choreography tools

To adapt the approach and add variety to the session use any of the following tools.

- Travel the movement, e.g. forwards, backwards, sideways, around in a small circle, facing all four sides of the room, in a big circle and moving inwards and out of the circle, diagonals, in lines etc.
- Combine different movements to form a sequence of movements – a pattern.
- Perform the movements at a different pace.
- Vary the speed within a sequence of moves.
- Vary the direction.
- Add a body movement, i.e. rib shift, hip wiggle, shoulder shrug, or another bodily gesture to add a more funky element to each basic move.
- Add arm lines.
- Use different arm lines within a sequence of moves.

# Summary of the guidelines for structuring the cardio-vascular component

## Re-warmer/build-up aerobics

- Start at a low intensity and progressively build to a higher intensity by bending deeper, jumping, and travelling further and more frequently.
- Spend longer on this component with less fit groups to allow for a more gradual increase of the heart rate.
- Spend less time on this component with fitter participants who are able to build up to working at a higher intensity more rapidly.

## Maintenance

- Use exercises which utilise the large muscle groups to demand greater volumes of oxygen and create the desired effect.
- Alter the stress on the joints by using a mixture of jumping, bending and travelling movements.
- Utilise less frequent and shorter bursts of higher intensity activities for less fit participants to enable them to work out safely and effectively.
- Utilise frequent and longer bursts of more intense activities for fitter participants to make their hearts work harder and to challenge their cardio-vascular system.
- Use jumping movements sparingly with less fit participants who have heavier body weights.
- Spend longer on this component with fitter participants.
- Spend comparatively less time on this component with less fit participants.

## Pulse-lowering/cool-down

- Start at a high intensity and progressively decrease the amount of jumping, travelling and depth of bending movements.
- Spend longer on this component with less fit participants, allowing them a longer time to recover.
- Spend less time on this component with fitter participants, who are generally able to recover more quickly.

# CARDIO-VASCULAR EXERCISES

| Ex 1 | Jumping jacks |
| --- | --- |

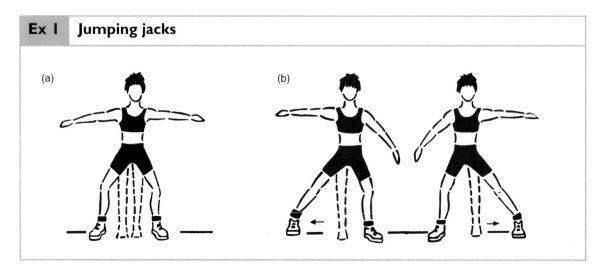

(a)

(b)

## Starting position and instructions

Stand with feet hip width apart. Bend the knees and push through the thigh muscles to jump the legs to a wider straddled position. Raise the arms outwards to the side of the body and in line with the shoulders as the legs jump outwards (*see* figure a). Jump the feet back together, bringing the arms down at the same time. Develop a rhythmic action.

## Teaching points

- Keep the knee joints unlocked.
- Ensure the heels go down when landing.
- Ensure the knees travel in line with the toes and over the ankles. Take care not to let the knees roll inwards.
- Keep the elbows slightly bent throughout the movement.
- Keep the abdominal muscles pulled in to avoid hollowing of the lower back.
- Keep the hips facing forwards and the back straight.

## Progressions

- To lower the impact, step the legs alternately out to the side without jumping (*see* figure b). The supporting knee must remain slightly bent and in line with the ankle. This exercise can be progressed by adding a jump in between each alternate leg lunge (becomes high impact when jumps added). Progressing to a higher jump and faster movement will increase the intensity considerably.
- Performing the Jumping Jacks at a slightly slower pace initially will lower the intensity.
- Increase the intensity by travelling the exercise forwards and backwards for either four or eight counts to move the resistance of the body across the force of gravity.
- Increase the intensity further by progressing to a Power Jack. To perform a Power Jack slow down the jumping out movement and bend deeper for two counts; return the legs back together by performing two small jumps for two counts.

## Ex 2 Jogging

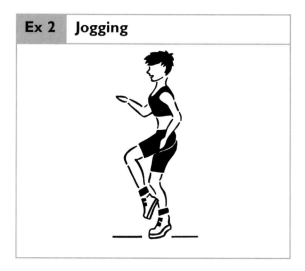

### Starting position and instructions

Starting with the feet hip width apart. Commence jogging alternate legs on the spot.

### Teaching points

- Ensure the heels go down to the floor as this will maximise movement through the ankle and will prevent the calf muscles cramping (aim for a ball of the foot through to the heel landing).
- Land lightly.
- Keep the knees unlocked and slightly soft throughout the movement.
- Keep the hips facing forwards, the back straight and abdominals pulled in.

- If the arms are used, ensure they move in a controlled fashion and that the elbows remain unlocked.
- If travelling the movement forwards, aim for a heel through to toe action of the foot to achieve a more natural running action.

### Progressions

- To lower the impact, march or walk on the spot. Note: it is essential that the feet land lightly if it is used as a low-impact exercise.
- Start at a steady pace and move through a small and lower range of motion with the feet lifting only slightly from the floor.
- Progressively move at a faster pace and through a larger range of motion. Moving the body's resistance upwards will increase the intensity of the movement.
- Vary the speed of the movement. Try slow jogs, where instead of using a single count, two counts are used for each foot strike. Alternatively, speed the movement up to a sprint pace, or use a combination of slow and fast time, i.e. slow, slow, quick, quick, slow for eight counts.
- Travel the movement forwards and backwards, or around in a small or large circle or figure of eight. Shifting the body weight across the force of gravity in this way will increase the intensity of the movement.

| Ex 3 | Spotty dogs |
| --- | --- |

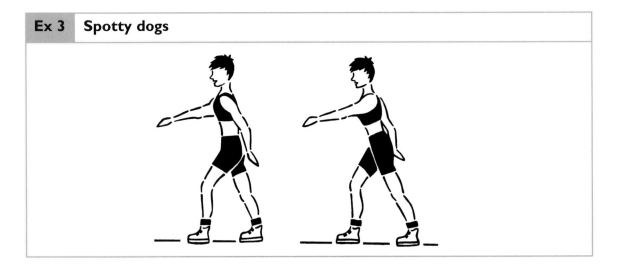

## Starting position and instructions

Stand with the feet hip width apart. Bend the knees and push through the thighs to stride the legs alternately backwards and forwards. Use the arms in opposition to the legs.

## Teaching points

- Try to ensure the heels go down to the floor. Care should be taken not to force the heel of the back leg to the floor, unless it feels comfortable. This could cause a ballistic stretch of the calf muscle, depending on the flexibility of the individual and the speed of the movement.
- Progressively stride the legs with a larger range of motion, but only move through a range of motion that feels comfortable.
- Keep the hips facing forwards and avoid hollowing of the lower back by tightening the abdominal muscles.
- Keep both knees unlocked. This will avoid placing any stress on the cruciate ligaments which help to stabilise the knee joint.
- If the arms are used, ensure all movements are controlled and keep the elbows unlocked.

## Progressions

- To lower the impact, step alternate legs backwards, keeping the weight-bearing knee slightly bent. Impact can be added and the intensity progressed in this variation by adding a jump in between the alternate steps. This increases the intensity considerably.
- Start with small strides and increase to a larger range of motion by increasing the stride distance.
- Move at a progressively faster pace.
- Vary the speed of the movement. Moving slower and bending the knees more will vary the movement to a Power Lunge and will increase the intensity. Alternatively, combining some slow- and quick-paced moves will vary the choreography, i.e. slow, slow, quick, quick, quick, quick for an eight-beat count.

## Ex 4    Gazelle leaps

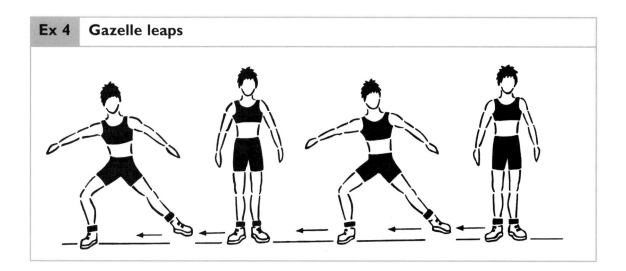

### Starting position and instructions

Stand with the feet hip width apart. Bend the knees and push through the thigh muscles to create an upwards and sideways travelling motion. Flick the toe of the trailing leg to execute the movement more gracefully. Travel for the desired number of repetitions in one direction and then repeat in the other direction.

### Teaching points

- Keep the knee joints unlocked.
- Ensure the heels go down and soften the knees when landing.
- Keep the hips facing forwards, the abdominals pulled in, the back straight and the chest lifted.

### Progressions

- To lower the impact, step the movement to the side rather than jumping. Decreasing the upwards movement of the body against the force of gravity will lower the intensity.
- To increase the intensity of lower impact movements take wider strides and bend deeper.
- When performing as a high-impact move, start with a small leap by pushing less forcefully through the thigh muscles.
- Progress to a larger leap, jumping higher and travelling further by exerting a greater force through the thighs.
- Travelling the movement more in one direction will increase the repetitions and require greater muscular endurance. It will also require more effort to shift the body weight across the force of gravity.

## Ex 5   Flick kicks (front, side and back)

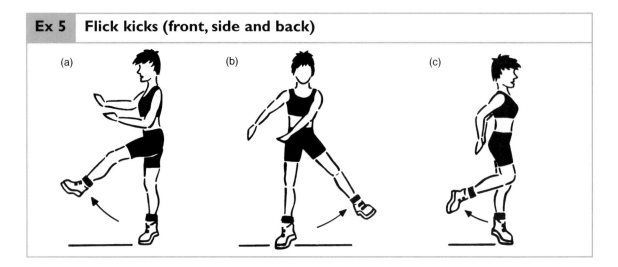

(a)  (b)  (c)

### Starting position and instructions

Stand with the feet hip width apart. Hop on the right leg and at the same time kick the left leg (a) forwards or (b) to the side or (c) backwards~j. Repeat this action, hopping on the left leg and kicking the right leg forwards or to the side or backwards.

### Teaching points

- Keep the weight-bearing knee joint un-locked.
- Take care not to lock the other knee as the leg kicks forwards, sideways or backwards.
- Ensure the heel goes down and soften the knee as the foot lands. Take care not to let the knee roll in.
- Keep the hips facing forwards and avoid hollowing of the lower back by keeping the abdominal muscles pulled in tight, the buttocks tucked in and the chest lifted.

### Progressions

- To lower the impact, perform the move without a hop (step and kick). Bend the knee of the weight-bearing leg to maintain some intensity.
- Start with a small hop and keep the kick low.
- Progress to a larger hop and a higher kick.
- Travel the movement forwards and/or backwards to shift the body weight across the force of gravity.
- Vary the speed of the movement by performing some slow and some quick kicks.
- Add variety by kicking the legs to the side of the body or behind the body.
- Perform a variety of front, side and back kicks as a movement sequence.
- Travel the movement and add a turn midway through a travelling sequence. For example, perform four forward travelling kicks and half turn the body on the third kick to face the back of the room and half turn the body on the fourth kick to face the front again.

## Ex 6 | Knee lifts

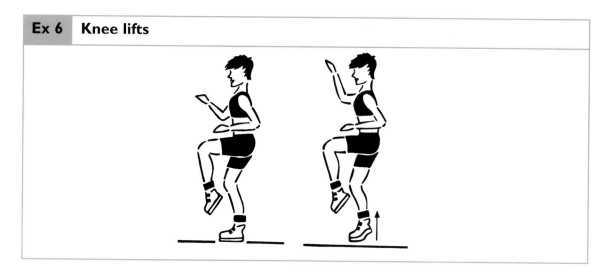

### Starting position and instructions

Start with the feet hip width apart. Hop on to the right leg and lift the left knee to hip height. Hop and transfer the weight to the left leg and lift the right knee to hip height.

### Teaching points

- Keep the knee of the weight-bearing leg slightly bent throughout the movement.
- Ensure the heels go down after jumping.
- Keep the hips facing forwards and avoid hollowing of the lower back by keeping the abdominal muscles pulled in.
- Keep the back straight and the chest lifted.

### Progressions

- Start by lifting the knees without a hop.
- Progress by adding a small hop, not lifting the body very high from the floor.
- Move at a progressively faster pace.
- Alternate the speed of movements – slow lift, slow lift, quick, quick, quick, quick.
- Alternate each knee lift to reduce muscular endurance.

- Perform two, four or eight lifts on the same side to increase muscular endurance.
- Travel the alternating knee lifts forwards and backwards.
- Travel the repetitive knee lifts sideways to the right or left.
- Turn in a small circle while performing the movement.
- Perform two alternating knee lifts and two repetitive knee lifts, i.e. right, left, right for two lifts, left, right, left for two knee lifts.
- Perform two knee lifts each side but take the leg behind the body on the first knee lift and back to the start position on the second. Repeat the same on the other side.
- Perform as above, but take the knee across the front of the body on the first knee lift and back to the start position on the second.
- Perform four knee lifts on each side, taking the first across the front, the second to return to centre, the third behind the back, the fourth back to centre. Repeat the same on the other side.

## Ex 7 | Pendulums

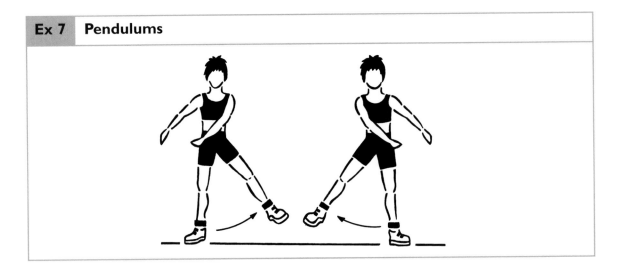

### Starting position and instructions

Stand with the feet hip width apart. Hop on to the right leg and at the same time kick the left leg out to the side, rocking and leaning the body towards the right. Repeat this action, hopping on to the left leg, kicking the right leg to the side and leaning the body towards the left. Develop a rocking, swinging type of motion.

### Teaching points

- Keep the weight-bearing knee joint unlocked.
- Ensure the heel goes down and soften the knee as the foot lands. Take care not to let the knee roll in.
- Keep the hips facing forwards and avoid hollowing of the lower back.
- Keep the abdominal muscles pulled in tight, the buttocks tucked in, the chest lifted and the shoulders back.

### Progressions

- To lower the impact, perform the move without a hop (step and side kick). Bend the knee of the weight-bearing leg to maintain some intensity.
- Start with a small hop and keep the kick low.
- Progress to a larger hop with a higher kick and more momentum.
- Travel the movement forwards and/or backwards to shift the body weight across the force of gravity.
- Vary the speed of the movement by performing some slow and some quick movements, i.e. rock, rock hold right, rock, rock hold left.
- Add variety by rocking the legs forwards and backwards instead of side to side.

## Ex 8    Gallops

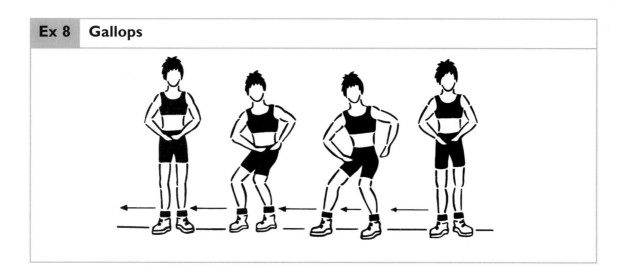

### Starting position and instructions

Stand with the feet hip width apart. Commence a sideways galloping movement to the right for the desired number of repetitions. Return to the starting position with the same movement to the left.

### Teaching points

- Keep the knees unlocked and slightly soft.
- Ensure the heel goes down as the foot lands – take care not to land only on the ball of the foot.
- Take great care not to let the knees roll in.
- Keep the hips facing forwards and avoid hollowing of the lower back.
- Keep the abdominal muscles pulled in tight, the buttocks tucked in, the chest lifted and the shoulders back.

### Progressions

- To lower the impact, walk to the side.
- Start with a small travelling distance and progressively travel further.
- Start at a slower pace.
- Progress by galloping with more momentum and pace.
- Perform a stationary movement before changing direction and returning to the start position.
- Add variety by galloping right (right leg leads) for two counts, pivot turning to face the back of the room and galloping in the same direction for a further two counts but with the left leg leading. Repeat to return to the front-facing start position.
- Perform the gallops in a box shape, i.e. gallop right for four, quarter pivot turn to face right; gallop left for four, quarter pivot turn to face the back; gallop right for four, quarter pivot turn to face left; gallop left for four, quarter pivot turn to face the front.

| Ex 9 | Pony |
|---|---|

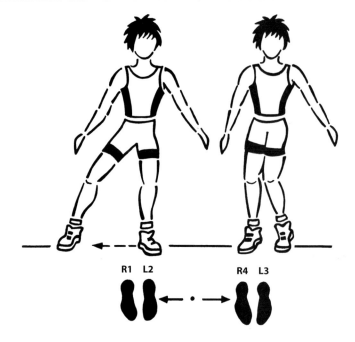

R1  L2        R4  L3

NB: Repeat on the opposite side, with a small jump.

## Starting position and instructions.

Start by stepping to the right and tapping the left leg in, repeat left. Build the step to a small jump to the right with a little ball change/run action of the feet.

For example:
Small jump to right side – right, left, right leg action (1 and 2 counts) small pause 2nd count. Repeat small jump to left side – left, right, left (3 and 4 counts) small pause on 4th count.

## Teaching points

• Heels down.
• Land lightly.
• Knees unlocked.

• Abdominals pulled in.
• Chest lifted.

## Progression/adaptation

• Increase height of the jump.
• Bring in an arm line to increase co-ordination.
• Travel the movement forwards and backwards.

## Ex 10 Heel raise/calf raise

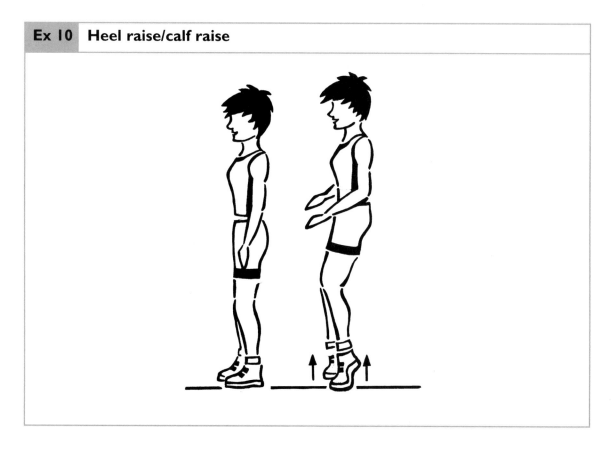

### Starting position and instructions

Start with your feet hip width apart. Raise onto the balls of the feet so that the heels lift off the floor rythmically.

### Teaching points

- Make sure the ankles do not roll outwards.
- Keep the balls of the feet on the floor.
- Knees unlocked.
- Abdominals pulled in.
- Chest lifted.

### Progression/adaptation

- Add a small jump so that the body lifts off the floor.
- Bring in an arm line to increase co-ordination.
- Turn the movement in a circle.
- Adapt by bending the knees instead of lifting heels.

## Ex II  Side lunge and back lunge

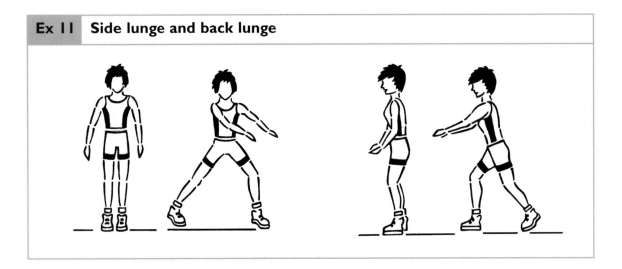

## Starting position and instructions

Start with the feet together:

**Side lunge:**
Keeping the left knee bent, lunge and tap the right leg out to the right side.
Repeat with the other leg.

**Back lunge:**
Keeping the left knee bent, lunge and tap the right leg backwards
Repeat with the other leg.

## Teaching points

• Support knee in line with toes and over ankles.
• Knees unlocked.
• Abdominals pulled in and hips face forward.
• Chest lifted.
• Heels down when impact added.

## Progression/adaptation

• Increase depth of bend on supporting leg
• Add a jump in between transitions to increase impact
• Bring in an arm line to increase co-ordination
• Increase repetitions. for example, double lunge right, double lunge left.
• Add a power jump off the supporting leg to transfer weight to other leg.

## Ex 12   Mambo

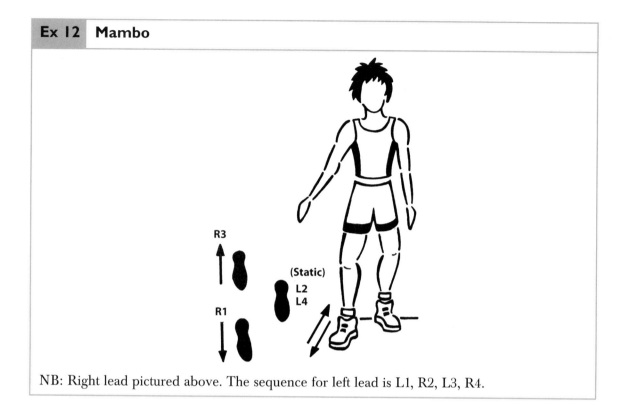

NB: Right lead pictured above. The sequence for left lead is L1, R2, L3, R4.

## Starting position and instructions

Start with the feet together
1. Step the right leg forward, taking the weight onto the right leg (count 1)
2. Return the weight to the left leg (count 2)
3. Step the right leg backwards, taking the weight onto the left leg (count 3)
4. Return the weight to the left leg.
To change legs: Repeat 1 and 2 THEN perform a ball change (run, run, run action – 3 counts) to enage left leg lead.

## Teaching points

- Weight bearing knee unlocked and in line with ankle.
- Abdominals pulled in and hips face forward.
- Chest lifted.
- Heels down when impact added.

## Progression/adaptation

- Add a jump in between transitions to increase impact.
- Bring in an arm line to increase co-ordination.
- Add a pivot turn in the movement sequence.
- Link with other choreography.

| Ex 13 | **Mambo and chasse** |
|---|---|

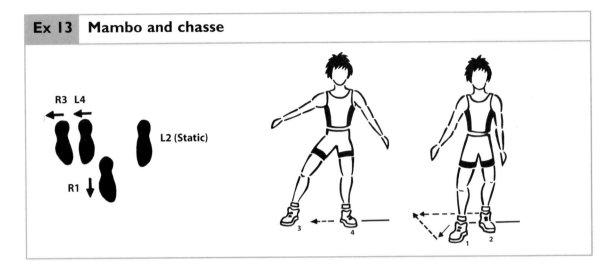

## Starting position and instructions

Start with the feet together:
1. Step the right leg forward, taking the weight onto the right leg (count 1)
2. Return the weight to the left leg (count 2)
3. Step right, step left leg together with right, step right (count 3 and 4)
4. Repeat left.

## Teaching points

- Weight bearing knee unlocked and in line with ankle.
- Abdominals pulled in and hips face forward.
- Chest lifted.
- Heels down on chasse.

## Progression/adaptation

- Travel chasse further by making move bigger.
- Add a jump in between transitions to increase impact.
- Bring in an arm line to increase co-ordination.

# ARMS LINES

| Ex 1 | Biceps curl |
|------|-------------|

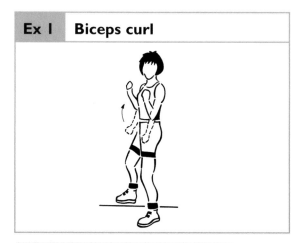

## Starting position and instructions

Keeping the elbows pressed into the sides of the body, raise the forearms and curl the hands towards the shoulders in an arc-like motion. Return the arms to the side without locking the elbows. Try with a squat.

| Ex 2 | Lateral raise |
|------|---------------|

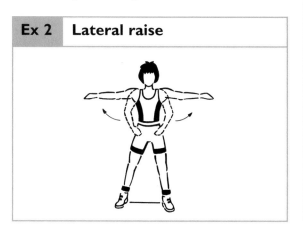

## Starting position and instructions

Start with the arms at the side of the body. Raise the arms sideways until they are at shoulder height. Keep the elbows unlocked and the shoulders relaxed and down. Try with side squats.

| Ex 3 | Breaststroke |
|------|--------------|

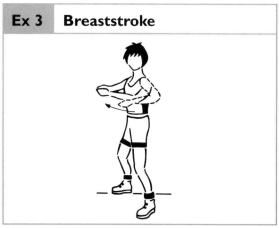

## Starting position and instructions

Move the arms in a breaststroke swimming action, either in front of the body or above the head. Keep the shoulders relaxed and the elbows unlocked. Try with a grapevine.

| Ex 4 | Shoulder press |
|------|----------------|

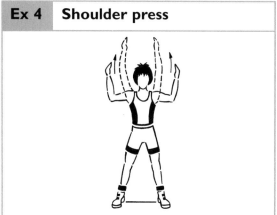

## Starting position and instructions

Start with the arms bent and the elbows level with the shoulders. Press the arms above the head and extend the arms, then return to the starting position. Keep the shoulders relaxed and the elbows unlocked. Try with knee lifts.

| **Ex 5** | **Front raise** |
|---|---|

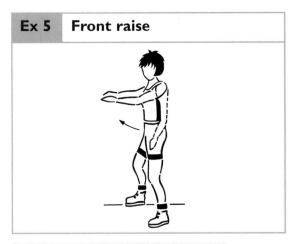

## Starting position and instructions

Start with the arms by the side of the body. Raise the arms in front of the body to shoulder height and lower. Keep the elbows slightly bent. Try with back lunge.

| **Ex 6** | **Pec dec** |
|---|---|

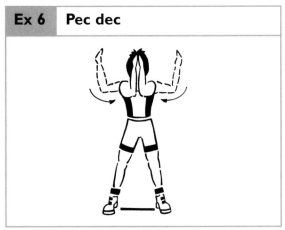

## Starting position and instructions

Start with the arms at shoulder height and the elbows bent, hands pointing upwards. Squeeze the arms together in front of the body and return to the side. Take care not to fling the arms too far back. Try with leg curls and knee lifts.

| **Ex 7** | **Criss cross diagonals** |
|---|---|

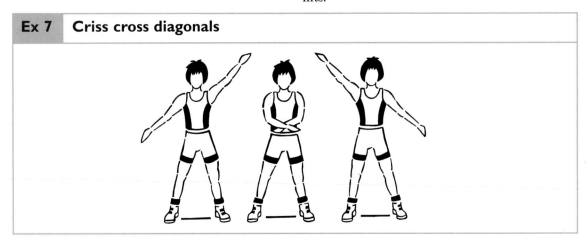

## Starting position and instructions

Start with the arms at the side of the body. Cross the arms in front of the body and then take the left arm up and to the left and the right arm down and to the right. Cross the arms in front of the body again, and this time take the left arm down towards the left and the right arm up towards the right. Take care not to fling the arms. Try with jogging.

| **Ex 8** | **Scissors** |
| --- | --- |

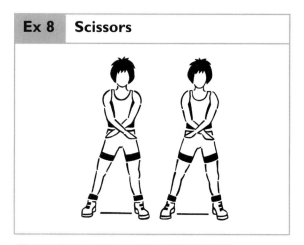

## Starting position and instructions

Scissor the arms in front of the body, either wide and slow, or small and fast scissors.

| **Ex 9** | **Waterfall** |
| --- | --- |

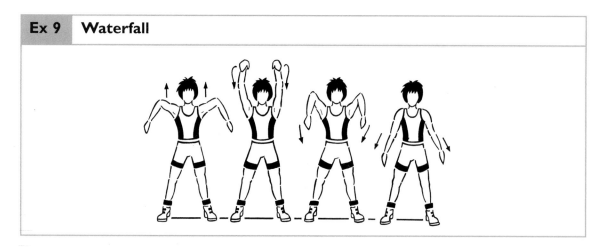

## Starting position and instructions

Raise the arms upwards and close to the body and extend them over the head. Ripple the arms down to form a waterfall effect as they lower to the starting position.

| Table 7.5 | General example of building up aerobic intensity (Mixed ability) | | |
|---|---|---|---|
| **Timing** | **Exercise Description and Purpose** | **Alternative** | **Progression** |
| **NB:** The whole programme is designed to accompany one song – adapt your timings accordingly | A<br>Double grapevine R and march<br>Double grapevine L and march | Side steps or walk and march | Add an arm line |
| | B<br>Walk forward and march<br>Walk backwards and march<br>Repeat. | | |
| | Repeat A<br>Replace march with back lunge | | Bend deeper and add an arm line |
| | Repeat B<br>Replace march with _ jump | | Bend deeper and add an arm line |
| | Repeat A<br>Replace back lunge with spotty dogs | Stay with back lunge but bend a little deeper | |
| | Repeat B<br>Jog forward and full jacks | Stay with walks and/or jacks but take longer stride and bend deeper | |
| | Repeat A | | |
| | Repeat B | | |

| Table 7.6 | General example of maintaining aerobic intensity (Mixed ability) | | |
|---|---|---|---|
| **Timing** | **Exercise Description and Purpose** | **Alternative** | **Progression** |
| **NB:** The whole programme is designed to accompany one song – adapt your timings accordingly | A<br>Scoop forwards × 4<br>Jog backwards × 4<br>Power jacks × 4<br>Repeat all above | Walk backwards with jacks | Deeper bends<br>Add arm line.<br>Jump higher and bend deeper. |
| | B<br>Gallop right × 4 and jump in a circle × 4<br>Repeat left<br>And repeat. | Walk instead of gallop<br>Jump in place without turn | Travel further |
| | C<br>Gazelle leaps × 4 to right diagonal<br>Calf raise × 4<br>Repeat to return back to centre<br>Repeat C to left diagonal | Move to right and not diagonal | Jump higher<br><br>Add arm line to calf raise. |
| | D<br>Leg curls single, single double | | Add jump<br>Add _ turn on double to face side of room then back to front. |
| | Repeat A B C D | | |

| Table 7.7 | General example of cooling down aerobic intensity (Mixed ability) | | |
|---|---|---|---|
| **Timing** | **Exercise Description and Purpose** | **Alternative** | **Progression** |
| **NB:** The whole programme is designed to accompany one song – adapt your timings accordingly | A<br>Scoop forwards × 4<br>Jog backwards × 8<br>Power jacks × 4<br>Repeat all above | Walk backwards or full jacks | Deeper bends<br>Add arm line<br>Jump higher and bend deeper. |
| | B<br>Double grapevine R and spotty dogs<br>Repeat L<br>Repeat B again | Back lunge but bend deeper | |
| | Repeat A but replace power jacks with full or _ jacks | Walk backwards and _ jacks | |
| | Repeat B but replace spotty dogs with back lunge | | |
| | Repeat A but walk back to replace jogs | | |
| | Repeat B but travel less on double grapevine | | |
| | Repeat A and B progressively | | |

# DESIGNING A STEP
# TRAINING PROGRAMME

## 8

Step training is an effective method of training to improve cardio-vascular fitness. The stepping action itself is low impact in nature, and the intensity of the workout is achieved by using the larger muscles of the lower body to shift the body weight (centre of gravity) from the ground, up on to the step and back down to the floor. Traditionally, methods for progressing a step class are to raise the step height and travel around and over the step more frequently throughout the session. These activities increase the range of motion through which the body is moving and are therefore more demanding and as a consequence more intense. However, as with other approaches, too much repetition of the same joint action can overstress the muscles and joints. Therefore, the movements used need to be sufficiently varied to provide a balanced workout.

Step training has evolved tremendously over recent years and many teachers have developed their own choreography, introducing jumping and propulsive movements on to and around the step. These activities are very effective ways of raising the intensity and provide greater opportunity for varying movements. However, they are high impact in nature. Therefore, to design a safe and effective step exercise to music programme the same safety principles as for other cardio-vascular training activities should be applied. Mixing the levels of impact and varying the approach to the step and joint actions are ways to reduce the occurrence of repetitive strain injuries and overstressed joints.

## How should an ETM step training session be structured?

ETM step sessions should follow the same structural design as any other session that targets cardio-vascular fitness. This is outlined in table 8.1.

Ideally, the step should be utilised in all components of the session to avoid any unnecessary disruptions to the flow of the class. Guidelines for using the step in each component are outlined in this chapter.

## How should the warm-up be adapted for an ETM step session?

It is essential to include use of the step in the warm-up component to orientate participants to the positioning of the step and familiarise them with basic movements. For fitter groups, movement patterns that will be used in the main workout can be introduced at a slower pace and lower intensity during the warm-up. This will allow for any specific skill advice to be provided. Less fit participants will not be able to cope with the intensity if the step is used too frequently in the warm-up. Low-intensity movements around the step, or marching on and off the step and tapping the step, will probably be more appropriate for orientating them to the step without raising the intensity too much.

| Table 8.1 | The structure of an ETM step training session |
|---|---|
| *Warm-up* | • Mobility and pulse-raising exercises.<br>• Preparatory stretches. |
| *Main workout (1): cardio-vascular training* | • Re-warmer/build-up aerobics to raise the intensity.<br>• Maintenance of intensity at an appropriate level.<br>• Pulse-lowering/cool-down exercises to lower intensity and promote venous return. |
| *Main workout (2): muscular strength and endurance training (optional)* | • Specific toning exercises for muscles not targeted in the main session (back, chest, abdominals, arms). |
| *Cool-down* | • Post-workout stretches (maintenance and developmental).<br>• Relaxation (optional).<br>• Re-mobilise. |

*Note*: If muscular strength and endurance exercises are included, the session will follow the traditional ETM session format and will include training all the components of fitness.

## How should the cardio-vascular training component be adapted for an ETM step session?

During the main workout the step should be used maximally. However, it is often a good idea to include some floor-based movements around the step to vary and alter the repetitive nature of continuous stepping.

The intensity should follow the traditional build-up, maintenance and build-down of levels as adopted in other cardio-vascular training sessions. The build-up can be achieved by gradually increasing the movement around and over the step. The build-down can be achieved by progressively reducing the movement over and around the step. It should be recognised that during the maintenance component, when new step patterns are introduced, the intensity may lower temporarily until the sequence is established and all participants are able to follow. For this reason, step exercise to music will tend to follow an interval training format, where the intensity is built up while adding together one sequence of exercises, and lowered again (slightly) while the second sequence of exercises is added and so forth. A fitter and more skilful group will tend to pick up each movement sequence more quickly. They will therefore spend less time learning and performing the sequence at a low intensity, and will spend more time performing the activity at the target high-intensity pace.

Step exercises are illustrated with instructions at the end of this chapter. These are followed by examples of step choreography.

## How should the muscular strength and endurance and post-workout stretching components be adapted for an ETM step session?

The steps can be removed prior to any muscular strength and endurance and post-workout stretching activities, however this needs to be managed effectively so that class flow is not interrupted too much. If the steps are removed, the traditional ETM muscular strength and endurance and post-workout stretching exercises can be performed. If the steps are not removed, it is appropriate to utilise the step in some way during these components.

The step can be used to enhance the effectiveness of some muscular strength and endurance activities by offering a greater range of motion for some exercises. Figure 8.1 illustrates four exercises where the range of motion or resistance are increased to raise the intensity. The step can also be used to assist the performance of certain stretches as illustrated in figure 8.2.

### Figure 8.1 Using the step to increase the intensity of muscular strength and endurance exercises

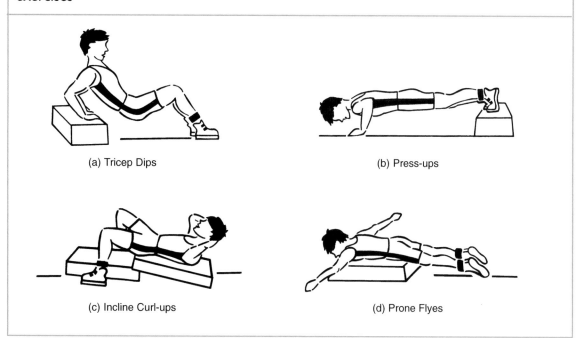

(a) Tricep Dips

(b) Press-ups

(c) Incline Curl-ups

(d) Prone Flyes

(a) **Tricep Dips** off the step provide a larger range of motion through which the body can move.
(b) **Press-ups**, by raising the feet or knees on to the step, elevate the weight of the body and provide more resistance for the muscles.
(c) **Incline Curl-ups** require the abdominal muscles to work through a larger range of motion against the resistance of gravity.
(d) **Prone Flyes** performed off the step provide a larger range of motion for the trapezius muscle to work through.

## Figure 8.2 Using the step for effective post-workout stretches

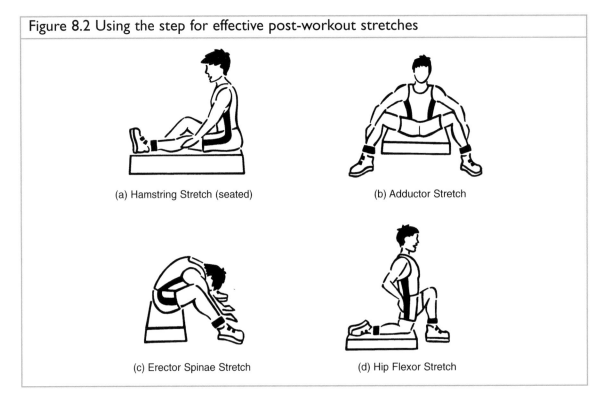

(a) Hamstring Stretch (seated)

(b) Adductor Stretch

(c) Erector Spinae Stretch

(d) Hip Flexor Stretch

(a) and (b) The **Hamstring and Adductor Stretches** performed on the step require less flexibility in the erector spinae muscles than would be required if seated on the floor. Therefore most participants are able to achieve an effective stretch of the muscles while in these positions.

(c) The **Erector Spinae Stretch** is performed more effectively in this position because sitting on a step does not require great levels of flexibility in the hamstring muscles.

(d) The **Hip Flexor Stretch** is much easier to perform by kneeling on the step. This position requires less flexibility of the hamstrings, gluteals and adductors in the weight-bearing leg so a more effective stretch is possible.

# STEP EXERCISES

**Ex I** | **Basic step/V step/Turn step**

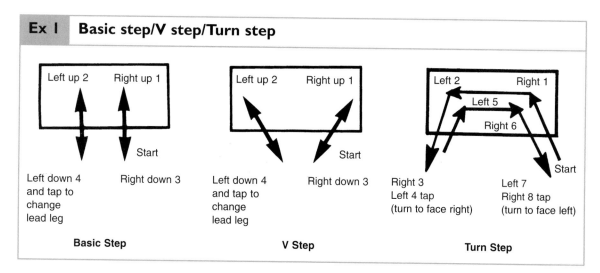

| Basic Step | V Step | Turn Step |

## Starting position

Stand on the floor with the feet hip width apart.

## Basic

Step on to the step leading with the right leg. Step back down to the floor again leading with the right leg. Tap to change to a left leg lead when desired.

## V Step

Step the feet out wide to each edge of the step. Right foot to right edge and left foot to left edge. Step the feet back down to the floor with the feet hip width apart (right foot, then left foot). Tap to change to a left leg lead.

## Turn Step

As for V Step above, but turn the body in the direction of the movement.

## Teaching points

- Keep the knee joints unlocked.
- Keep the back straight and abdominals pulled in.

- Keep the hips facing forwards and fully extend the hip and knee.
- Place the whole foot on the step and stay close to the step.
- Keep the knees in line with the toes. Take care not to let the knees roll inwards.
- Turn Step only: turn the body prior to placing the foot on the step to avoid strain on the knee.

## Progressions

- Start with slow time movement.
- Progress by working to normal time.
- Progress further by making each movement a run up on to the step.
- Use different arm lines to add variety.
- Add a floor-based movement in between each complete cycle of a movement to add variety.
- Jump to and hold the legs in the V Step position (two counts) and step down to perform as a power move which adds impact and intensity.

## Ex 2 | Up and tap/knee/curl/raise side/glut raise

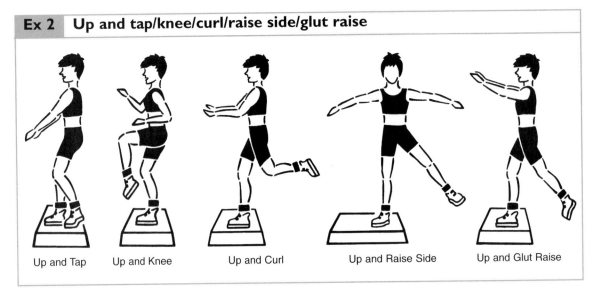

Up and Tap | Up and Knee | Up and Curl | Up and Raise Side | Up and Glut Raise

### Starting position

Stand on the floor with both feet hip width apart.

### Up and Tap

Step the right foot on to the step and tap the step with the left leg, step down left, down right. Repeat with the left leg leading.

### Up and Knee

As above, but lift the knee to hip height instead of tapping the step.

### Up and Curl

As above, but curl the heel towards the buttocks.

### Up and Raise Side

As above, but take the leg out towards the side.

### Up and Glut Raise

As above, but take the leg behind.

### Teaching points

- Keep the knee joints unlocked.
- Keep the back straight and abdominals pulled in.
- Keep the hips facing forwards and fully extend the hip and knee.
- Place the whole foot on the step and stay close to the step.
- Keep the knees in line with the toes. Take care not to let the knees roll inwards.

### Progressions

- Start with slow time movement, progress by working up to normal time.
- Use different arm lines to add variety.
- Perform a combination of the movements to challenge motor skills.
- Add a floor-based movement between each complete cycle of a movement to add variety.
- Travel the movement to each corner of the step.
- Travel the movement and perform two or more repetitions to each corner with a tap down in between.
- At one side perform three consecutive up and taps (or variation), i.e. up tap, up tap, up tap down, down to change legs and move to other side, repeat to complete the cycle. Repeating seven times will increase muscular endurance.

## Ex 3    Straddle step

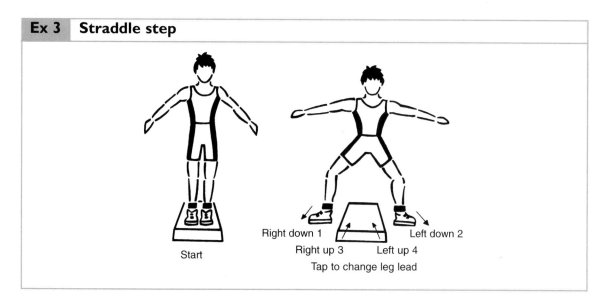

Start

Right down 1    Left down 2
Right up 3    Left up 4
Tap to change leg lead

## Starting position and instructions

Stand on top of the step. Step the right leg down to the side of the step, and then the left leg to stand, straddling the step. Step the right leg back up on to the step and follow with the left leg. Tap with the left leg to change to a left leg lead. As a variation to the tap up perform a Knee Raise/Leg Curl/Side Leg Raise/Glut Raise, as illustrated in exercise 2.

## Teaching points

- Ensure the feet are placed in the centre of the step.
- Ensure the whole foot lands on the step.
- Keep the knees in line with the toes and over the ankles.
- Keep the hips facing forwards.
- Keep the abdominals pulled in to avoid hollowing the lower back.

## Progressions

- Perform slow time and progressively build up to normal time.
- Perform with the smaller levers, i.e. tap up rather than knee up.
- Step down but jump up to perform as a power move.
- Perform a combination of straddles with varying leg moves (Knee Up × 2/Curl-Up × 2/Side Raise × 2/Power × 2). Lunges can be added to follow this sequence.

## Ex 4   Side lunges and rear lunges

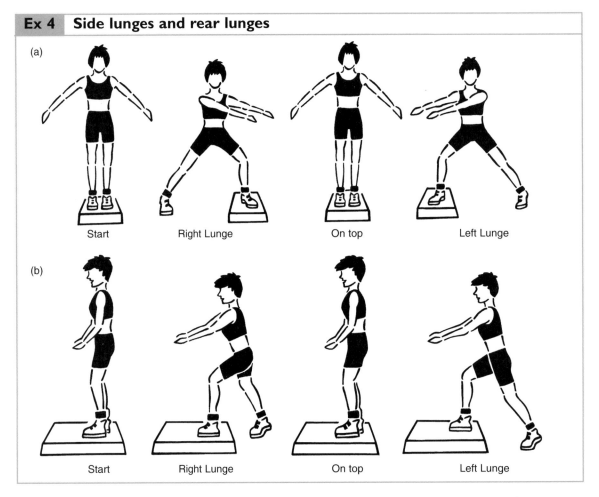

(a)

Start     Right Lunge     On top     Left Lunge

(b)

Start     Right Lunge     On top     Left Lunge

### Starting position and instructions

Stand on top of the step. Lunge alternate legs off the step, either (a) out to each side or (b) off the back.

### Teaching points

- Keep the knee joint unlocked and the whole foot on the step.
- Keep the back straight and the abdominals pulled in.
- Keep the knee in line with the toe and over the ankle, not letting the knee roll in.
- Keep the hips facing forwards.

- Tap the floor with the toe only. Do not transfer the weight of the body on to the lunging leg.

### Progressions

- Start with a small lunge, just tapping the foot.
- Progress by adding a rebound and jump between each lunge.
- Move at a slightly faster pace.
- Vary the speed, e.g. slow lunge, slow lunge, and four quick lunges.
- Perform more repetitions on the same leg to increase muscular endurance.

## Ex 5    Zig zag or Z step

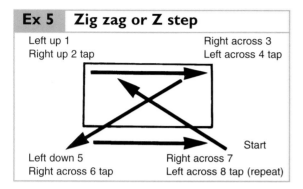

Left up 1
Right up 2 tap

Right across 3
Left across 4 tap

Start

Left down 5
Right across 6 tap

Right across 7
Left across 8 tap (repeat)

## Ex 6    W step

Right lead                    Left lead other side of box

5, 6        5, 6

1, 2        1, 2

3, 4                                    3, 4

Start

7, 8        7, 8

### Starting position and instructions

Stand facing the step with the feet shoulder width apart. Step the left leg to the left corner of the step and draw the right leg in towards it and tap the right foot. Step the right leg towards the right side of the step and draw the left leg in and tap. Step the left leg on to the floor to the left side and draw the right leg in and tap. Step the right leg to the right side and draw the left leg in and tap.

### Teaching points

- Keep the knee joints unlocked.
- Ensure the whole foot lands on the step.
- Keep the hips facing forwards.
- Keep the back straight and the abdominals pulled in.
- Take care not to let the knees roll in.

### Progressions

- Start with a small step and progress to larger steps.
- Add a jump on to the step.
- Add lunges to the sequence, e.g. up tap (R/L – 1, 2), lunge, lunge (L/R – 3, 4, 5, 6), side tap (L/R – 7, 8), lunge, lunge (R/L – 1, 2, 3, 4), down tap (L/R – 5, 6), side tap (L/R – 7, 8).
- Step off the front of the step instead of the back to vary the movement, ensuring the knees travels in line with the toes.
- Use different arm lines.
- Combine with another movement to form a sequence.

### Starting position and instructions

Stand in a straddle position facing the step. Step the right foot on to the right corner of the step and tap the left leg up (1, 2). Step the left leg off to the left side of the step and tap the right foot to the floor off the step (3, 4). Step the right leg back on to the side of the step and tap the left leg on the step (5, 6). Step the left leg down and right leg down (7, 8). Repeat as above but with a left leg lead and moving to the left corner and side of the step.

### Teaching points

- Keep the whole foot on the step and fully extend the knee and hip.
- Keep the hips facing forwards.
- Keep the knees unlocked.
- Stay close to the step.

### Progressions

- Start at a slow pace and progressively move at a faster pace.
- Use different arm lines.
- Add a Knee Lift or another leg movement on the trailing leg as you step to the side and off the step.
- Add a Side Leg Raise or another leg movement on the trailing leg when returning to the top of the step from the side of the step.

## Ex 7 | Power squats

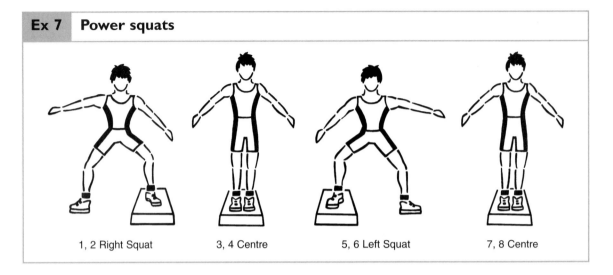

| 1, 2 Right Squat | 3, 4 Centre | 5, 6 Left Squat | 7, 8 Centre |

### Starting position and instructions

Stand on top of the step. Commence by stepping one leg out to the side into a squatting position, the other leg staying in contact with the step. Push through the thigh and lift the body back on to the step into the starting position. Repeat on the other side.

### Teaching points

- Squat the legs to a comfortable range of motion.
- Ensure the knees move in line with the toes and over the ankles.
- Do not let the knees roll inwards.
- Keep the hips facing forwards and avoid hollowing the lower back.
- Avoid locking the knee as the leg straightens.
- Keep the abdominals pulled in.
- Keep the whole foot on the step.

### Progressions

- Start with a small and slow movement.
- Progressively move at a faster pace and make the movement larger.
- Perform more repetitions on each side to increase muscular endurance.
- Perform a specified number of Squats and then Side Lunges.
- Use different arm lines
- Add a Leg Raise, Leg Curl or Knee Lift in between each Squat.

# CHOREOGRAPHY TOOLS

The principles for varying step choreography are similar to those used for basic cardio-vascular exercise. To add variety to step choreography use any of the following tools.

- Approach the step from a different position (from the front, from the side, from the top).
- Travel the movements (sideways over the top of the step – narrow or long end, diagonally forwards over the step, backwards or forwards along the side of the step, around the step, to diagonal corners of the step, pivot turn (quarter or half over the step)).
- Perform individual movements at different speeds.
- Vary the pace of each movement within a sequence.
- Add a body movement, i.e. rib shift, hip wiggle, shoulder shrug or another bodily gesture to add a more funky element to each Basic Step move.
- Add and use different arm lines.
- Combine different movements together to form a new sequence of movements – a new pattern (*see* examples provided).

## Examples of step choreography

### Basic Step/Pivot Turn/Straddle Step

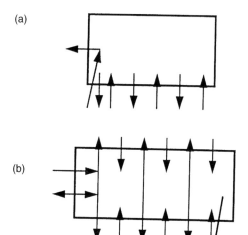

*Note*: the moves are in eight counts. Teaching points are the same as those for the Basic Step and Straddle Step. For the pivot turn add a hop to the movement to avoid twisting the knee joint.

### Instructions (a)

Perform three Basic Steps with a right leg lead, travelling along the step from right to centre to left:

    R up L up R down L down × 3
    1    2    3      4

Step up with the right leg and lift the left knee, hopping and pivot turning a quarter to face the left narrow side of the step:

    R up hop turn L knee lift
    5            6

Step off the narrow end – left leg – right leg;

    L down  R down.
    7       8

## Instructions (B)

Step on to the step with a left leg lead and and perform three straddle steps travelling forwards.

L up R up L down R down ¥ 3, travelling forwards

  1    2    3      4

On the last straddle, step left on to the step and hop on the left, pivot turning to return to the front:

L hop and quarter turn R down L down
  5 , 6             7      8

## T step

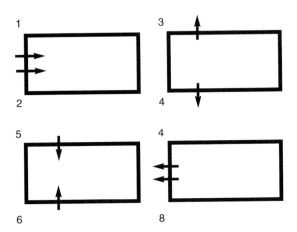

## Instructions

Face the narrow end of the step. Perform a Basic Step with a right leg lead on to the step (right up 1, left up 2). Straddle Step down from the step with a right leg lead (right down 3, left down 4). Straddle step up on to the step with a right leg lead (right up 5, left up 6). Basic Step down from the step with a right leg lead (right down 7, left down 8 or tap the left to change legs).

## Variations

Complete steps 1, 2, 3, 4 (basic up and straddle down) and replace steps 5 to 8 with a jump back movement to the start position. The legs will be straddling the step as the jumping back is performed. Alternatively, instead of jumping back, march back.

Step choreography has developed hugely in recent years. It is recommended that teachers attend training courses, workshops and master classes to broaden their awareness of these developments.

# DESIGNING A MUSCULAR STRENGTH & ENDURANCE TRAINING PROGRAMME

## How should a muscular strength and endurance training session be structured?

Specific muscular strength and endurance exercises are often included as a secondary workout in most ETM sessions. An appropriate session structure illustrating this format can be found in chapter 7, table 7.1. However, some ETM sessions devote the whole of the main workout to these two components of fitness. Body sculpt, body conditioning and new body classes are examples of ETM sessions where the sole emphasis is on improving the muscular strength and muscular endurance components of fitness. An appropriate structure for these specific types of sessions is outlined in table 9.1.

This chapter provides guidelines for structuring the muscular strength and endurance

component, whether as the secondary or main workout. It also illustrates a range of exercises for the major muscle groups. The benefits of training to improve muscular strength and endurance are discussed in chapter 1.

## What type of muscle work is most appropriate?

Exercises that require the specific muscles and muscle groups to contract and work through a full range of motion (isotonic movements) are most effective. Exercises that require the muscles to contract through a smaller range of motion, or those which require the muscle to contract without the muscle lengthening and shortening (isometric contractions) are less effective. Some of the advantages and disadvantages of these two types of muscle work are outlined in table 9.2.

| Table 9.1 | The structure of a muscular strength and endurance training session |
| --- | --- |
| *Warm-up* | • Mobility and pulse-raising exercises.<br>• Preparatory stretches.<br>• Re-warmer. |
| *Muscular strength and endurance training* | • Specific toning exercises targeting all major muscle groups to achieve a balanced whole body approach (with or without equipment). |
| *Cool-down* | • Cooling-down exercises.<br>• Post-workout stretches (inclusion of developmental stretches will improve flexibility).<br>• Relaxation (optional).<br>• Re-mobilise. |

| Table 9.2 | Advantages and disadvantages of isotonic and isometric muscle work |
|---|---|
| *Isotonic muscle work* | *Isometric muscle work* |
| Strengthens the muscle through a full range of motion. | Strengthens the muscle in one position only. |
| Closely related to our daily activities. | Most appropriate when moving the joint would create injury (i.e. injury rehabilitation). |
| Requires the recruitment of a large proportion of muscle fibres and nerves. | Requires the recruitment of the specific muscle fibres only to hold the position. |
| | Can potentially elevate blood pressure. |
| | Can cause participants to hold their breath. |

## How should we train to improve muscular strength and endurance?

To improve muscular endurance, it will be necessary to work the muscles for longer (high number of repetitions) with a lower resistance to movement. To improve muscular strength, it will be necessary to create further resistance to movement so that fewer repetitions of the activity can be performed. This can be achieved most easily by using external resistances such as bands, barbells and dumbbells. Gravity and extending body levers will also add some resistance to the exercises. Training methods to improve muscular strength and endurance are discussed in greater detail in chapter 1. A range of appropriate exercises to work the individual muscles are outlined in table 9.3. A series of resistance exercises, including exercises using barbells and dumbbells, clean-based lifts and bench lifts, are illustrated with step-by-step instructions at the end of this chapter. The exercises using external resistances can be used to design a body sculpt session and a sample lesson plan is provided on page 140.

| Table 9.3 | Joint actions when the major muscle groups contract concentrically and examples of exercises to work the muscles | | | |
|---|---|---|---|---|
| Muscle name | Anatomical position | Joints crossed | Prime action when contracting concentrically | Exercise |
| Gastrocnemius | Calf muscle | Knee and ankle | Plantarflexion – pointing the toe or rising on to the ball of the foot | Calf Raise (page 138) |
| Soleus | Calf muscle | Ankle | As above – with knee bent | Calf Raise with the knees bent |
| Tibialis anterior | Front of shin bone | Ankle | Dorsiflexion of the ankle – lifting the toe up towards the knee with the heel on the floor | Toe tapping |
| Hamstrings | Back of the thigh | Knee and hip | Flexion of the knee – lifting the heel towards the buttocks | Leg Curl (page 51) |
| Quadriceps | Front of the thigh | Knee and hip | Extension of the knee – straightening the knee | Back Squat (page 143) Dumbbell Lunge (page 139) Dead Lift (page 136) |
| Gluteus maximus | Buttock | Hip | Extension of the hip – lifting the leg out straight behind the body | Rear Leg Raise (page 131) Dead Lift Dumbbell Lunge |
| Iliopsoas (hip flexor) | Front hip | Hip | Flexion of the hip – lifting the knee to the chest | Knee Lift (page 95) |
| Abductors | Outside of hip and thigh | Hip | Abduction of the leg – taking the leg out to the side of the body | Side Leg Raise (page 129) |
| Adductors | Inside thigh | Hip | Adduction of the hip – taking the leg across the front of the body | Inner Thigh Raise (page 130) |

| Table 9.3 | Joint actions when the major muscle groups contract concentrically and examples of exercises to work the muscles cont. | | | |
|---|---|---|---|---|
| Muscle name | Anatomical position | Joints crossed | Prime action when contracting concentrically | Exercise |
| Rectus abdominus | Abdominals (front) | Spine | Flexion of the spine – bending the spine forwards | Sit-up/Curl-up Reverse Curl (page 126) |
| Erector spinae | Back of spine | Spine | Extension of the spine – straightening the spine | Back Extension (page 134) |
| Obliques | Side of trunk | Spine | Lateral flexion and rotation of the spine – twisting and bending the trunk to the side | Twisting Sit-up (page 127) |
| Pectorals | Front of the chest | Shoulder | Adduction and horizontal flexion of the arm – crossing the arms in front of the body | Press-up (page 133) Bench Press (page 146) Bent Arm Pull-over (page 147) Lying Dumbbell Flye (page 149) |
| Trapezius | Upper and middle back | Shoulder girdle | Extension of the neck – keeping the head up Elevation of the shoulder – lifting and lowering the shoulders Retraction of the scapula – squeezing the shoulder blades together | Upright Row (page 137) Prone Flye (page 135) |
| Latissimus | Side of the back | Shoulder | Adduction of the shoulder – drawing the arms down across the body or rowing movements of the arm | Single Arm Row (page 150) Bent Arm Pullover (page 147) |

| Table 9.3 | Joint actions when the major muscle groups contract concentrically and examples of exercises to work the muscles cont. | | | |
|---|---|---|---|---|
| Muscle name | Anatomical position | Joints crossed | Prime action when contracting concentrically | Exercise |
| Deltoids | Top of the shoulder | Shoulder | Abduction of the shoulder – lifting the arms out to the side of the body | Dumbbell Lateral Raise (page 141) Behind Neck Press (page 144) |
| Biceps | Front of the upper arm | Elbow and shoulder | Flexion of the elbow – bending the elbow | Barbell Curl (page 140) |
| Triceps | Back of the upper arm | Elbow and shoulder | Extension of the elbow – straightening the elbow | Press-up Tricep Dip Lying Tricep Extension Behind Neck Press Tricep Kickback |

*Note:* (1) This table has been adapted from *The Complete Guide to Exercise in Water*. It is designed to simplify the actions of the major muscles. Texts that provide a more detailed and descriptive analysis of muscular work are suggested in 'References and Recommended Reading' at the end of this book. (2) The named exercises will bring about both concentric (lifting phase of the movement) and eccentric (lowering phase of the movement) muscle contractions (isotonic muscle work).

## Summary of the guidelines for muscular strength and endurance training

To improve muscular endurance – perform more repetitions of the exercise.
To improve muscular strength – add further resistance to movement.

Add resistance by:

- increasing the range of motion
- decreasing the speed of the exercise
- increasing the leverage
- adding external resistance using bands, barbells, dumbbells, ankle weights, partner work.

Make the component harder by:

- increasing component time so more muscles can be worked, or a variety of exercises for the same muscle group can be included
- working the same muscle/muscle group more than once (multiple sets)
- working more muscles.

*Note:* whether strength or endurance is improved will depend on the number of repetitions one can perform. Lower rep ranges (1–10) will primarily improve strength; higher rep ranges (15–30) will primarily improve endurance; mid rep ranges (10–15) will improve both to some degree.

# RESISTANCE EXERCISES TO IMPROVE MUSCULAR STRENGTH AND ENDURANCE

| Ex 1 | Sit-ups/Curl-ups |
|---|---|

Hands on thighs

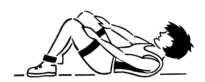

Hands across chest

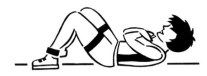

Hands side of head

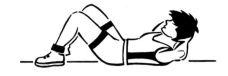

*Note:* correct breathing is essential when performing muscular strength and endurance exercises, especially the more strenuous exercises. The crucial point is that the breath is not held. Ideally, all outward breaths should occur on the effort – the lifting phase of the movement; inward breaths should occur on the lowering phase of the movement.

Hands above head

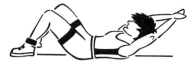

Crunch

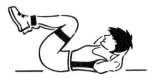

*Note:* The Crunch can be performed with the arms in any of the other positions.

## Purpose

This exercise will work the abdominal muscles at the front of the trunk (the rectus abdominus).

## Starting position and instructions

Lie on your back with your knees bent and your feet placed firmly on the floor. Tighten the abdominal muscles and pull them towards the back bone. Maintain this fixed position of the abdominals throughout the movement. Place your hands either on the thighs (easiest), across your chest (slightly harder), at the side of the head (harder still), or lengthen the arms above the head (hardest).

Contract the abdominal muscles to lift and curl the shoulders and chest upwards. Lift as far as is comfortable, but without lifting the lower back off the floor. Reverse the movement, keeping it controlled.

## Teaching points

- Tighten the abdominal muscles.
- Initiate the movement by contracting the abdominals and lifting the shoulders.
- Take care not to hollow the back; keep the back fixed.
- Keep the neck relaxed and look forwards, following the movement of the rest of the spine.
- Control the movement upwards and downwards.
- If the hands are placed at the side of the head do not pull on the head.

## Progressions

- Start with the shorter leverage positions, explained above, and progress to the longer leverage positions.
- Start with a regular pace of movement and progressively decrease the speed, for example take two counts to lift and two counts to lower.
- Progressively perform more repetitions to increase muscular endurance.
- External resistance can be placed across the chest to challenge muscular strength.
- A variation can be to lift the legs in the air and cross the ankles (a Crunch).
- A full Sit-up can be performed, however this will involve work of the hip flexor muscle and great care should be taken not to allow the back to hollow and hyperextend.

---

| Ex 2 | Twisting sit-ups |
| --- | --- |

Hands at side of head

Crunch

*Note:* the various lever positions illustrated in exercise 1 are equally appropriate for altering the intensity of this exercise.

## Purpose

This exercise will work the abdominal muscles at the side of the trunk (the obliques). It will also work the muscles at the front of the trunk (the rectus abdominus).

## Starting position and instructions

Lie on your back with your knees bent and your feet placed firmly on the floor. Tighten the abdominal muscles and pull them towards the back bone. Maintain this fixed position of the abdominals throughout the movement. Place your hands either on the thighs (easiest), across your chest (slightly harder), at the side of the head (harder still), or lengthen the arms above the head (hardest). Contract the abdominal muscles to lift and curl the shoulders and chest upwards, twisting the body to one side. Lower down and repeat this twisting to the other side.

## Teaching points

- Tighten the abdominal muscles.
- Initiate the movement by contracting the abdominals and lifting the shoulders.
- Take care not to hollow the back; keep the back fixed.
- Keep the neck relaxed and look forwards, following the movement of the rest of the spine.
- Control the movement upwards and downwards.
- If the hands are placed at the side of the head do not pull on the head.
- Lift only as far as is comfortable, but without lifting the lower back off the floor.
- Reverse the movement, keeping it controlled.
- Ease the shoulder towards the knee, rather than pulling the head over too far.

## Progressions

- Start with the shorter leverage positions explained above, and progress to the longer leverage positions.
- Start with a regular pace of movement and progressively decrease the speed, for example take two counts to lift and two to lower, or four counts to lift and four to lower.
- Progressively perform more repetitions to increase muscular endurance. Performing more repetitions on the same side will require greater endurance than alternating the lifts.
- A variation can be to lift the legs in the air and cross the ankles (a crunch).
- Cycling the legs can provide further variation, however care must be taken not to twist too far, or take the legs too low: lowering the legs too far will place unnecessary stress on the lower back.
- Lift one leg and draw pelvis towards you as you reach to the knee.

| Ex 3 | Reverse curls |
| --- | --- |

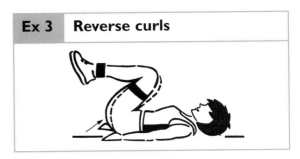

## Purpose

This exercise will work the muscles at the front of the trunk (the rectus abdominus).

## Starting position and instructions

Lie on the back. Lift the knees towards the chest so that they are in line with the bellybutton. Keep the knees slightly bent, or extend the legs, whichever is most comfortable. Tilt the pelvis to lift the buttocks from the floor so the knees move closer to the chest.

## Teaching points

- Initiate the movement from the abdominals.
- Tighten the abdominal muscles.
- Take care not to swing the legs.
- Take care not to hollow the lower back when returning the movement.
- Do not allow the legs to travel too far away from the central line of the body as this will place too much stress on the back.

## Progressions

- Perform the exercise at a slower pace so that the muscles have to contract and work for longer.
- As a variation, twist the legs towards the right shoulder and then the left shoulder to introduce some work for the oblique muscles.
- Combine the exercise with a Curl-up (illustrated in exercise 1) to increase the motor skills and muscle work involved.
- Vary the speed of the exercise, for example two slow double time and four normal pace.

| Ex 4 | Side leg raises |
|---|---|

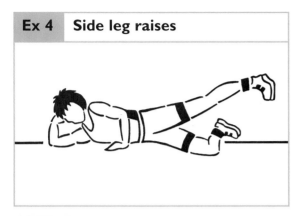

## Purpose

This exercise will work the muscles at the side of the hip, the abductors.

## Starting position and instructions

Lie on one side with the body in a straight line. Bend the lower knee to assist balance if necessary. Raise the top leg as high as you can, maintaining a straight spine with the hips in line with one another. Lower the leg, keeping the movement controlled. Continue for the desired number of repetitions.

## Teaching points

- Raise the leg with a controlled movement.
- Keep the abdominals pulled in tight.
- Take care not to swing the legs.
- Take care not to hollow the lower back or allow the hip to roll backwards.
- Keep a space between the hips and the ribs, and avoid swinging the trunk.

## Progressions

- Perform the exercise at a slow pace so that the muscles have to contract and work for longer.
- Vary the speed of the exercise, for example two slow double time and four normal pace.
- Perform through different ranges of motion, i.e. halfway up and down, all the way up and halfway down, up again and all the way down, all the way up and down.
- Perform a knee to chest movement, or Leg Curl in between each Side Leg Raise for variety.
- Perform standing to reduce the resistance of gravity to the movement by stepping and raising leg to the side.

## Ex 5 | Inner thigh raises

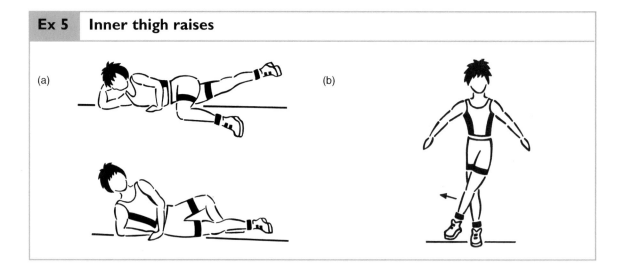

(a)

(b)

### Purpose

This exercise will work the muscles inside the thigh (the adductors).

### Starting position and instructions

Lie on one side with the body in a straight line, the upper arm on the floor and the head resting on the hand. Bend the top leg and either (a) rest it on the floor in front of the body, or (b) place it behind the straight leg with the foot on the floor if it is more comfortable. (If using the latter position take care not to let the hips roll backwards and make sure the knee is comfortable and not twisting.) Raise the lower leg as high as you can while maintaining a straight spine. Lower down under control. Perform for the desired number of repetitions.

### Teaching points

- Raise the leg under control.
- Keep the abdominals pulled in tight.
- Keep the movement controlled.
- Keep the spine straight.

### Progressions

- Perform the exercise at a slow pace so that the muscles have to contract and work for longer.
- Vary the speed of the exercise, e.g. two slow double time and four normal pace.
- Rest the foot of the upper leg on the thigh to add resistance and push down against the thigh to add further resistance to the movement.
- Perform standing up by crossing the leg over in front of the body to reduce the resistance of gravity to the movement. Note: to increase stability hold on to a wall.

## Ex 6 | Rear leg raises

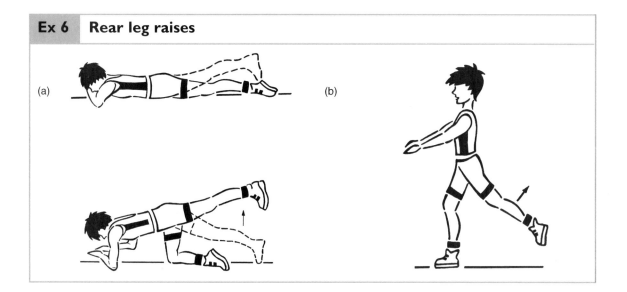

(a)

(b)

## Purpose

This exercise will work the buttock muscles (the gluteus maximus).

## Starting position and instructions

Lie face down on the floor (a), or kneel (b), as illustrated above. Raise one leg to just above hip height, ensuring that a straight spine is maintained. Lower the leg, keeping the movement controlled. Continue for the desired number of repetitions.

## Teaching points

- Raise the leg with a controlled movement.
- Keep the abdominals pulled in tight, and take care not to hollow the back.
- Take care not to swing the leg.
- If kneeling, take care not to rest on the knee cap or roll the body weight too far over to one side.
- If lying, keep the hip bones pressed towards the floor and lift the bellybutton towards the back bone.

## Progressions

- Perform the exercise at a slow pace so that the muscles have to contract and work for longer.
- Vary the speed of the exercise, for example two slow double time and four normal pace.
- Perform through different ranges of motion, i.e. halfway up and down, all the way up and halfway down, up again and all the way down, all the way up and down.
- Perform a knee to chest movement, or Leg Curl, in between each Rear Leg Raise for variety.
- Perform standing to reduce the resistance of gravity to the movement by stepping forward on one leg and raising rear leg behind body.

## Ex 7    Tricep dips

*Note:* these positions show methods of progressively increasing the intensity.

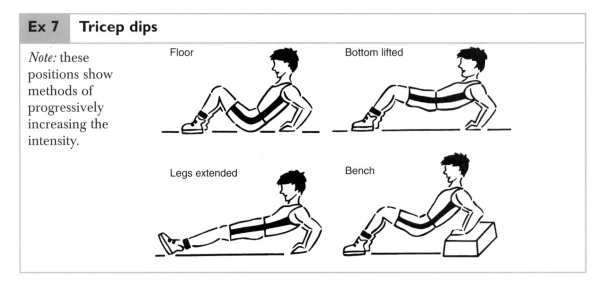

Floor

Bottom lifted

Legs extended

Bench

## Purpose

This exercise will work the muscles at the back of the upper arms (the triceps).

## Starting position and instructions

Sit on the floor with the knees bent and the feet flat on the floor. Position the hands about 12 inches behind the buttocks with the fingers pointing towards the body. Bend and straighten the elbows to lift and lower the body weight. Continued for the desired number of repetitions.

## Teaching points

- Raise and lower the body under control.
- Keep the abdominals pulled in tight and take care not to hollow the back.
- Ensure the elbows extend fully as the body is lifted up, but do not lock the elbows.
- If the buttocks are lifted off the floor, ensure the body is fixed and only the elbows move.
- If the legs are extended, take care not to lock the knee joint.
- On the bench, check that the elbows bend and the body lowers to a comfortable range of motion.

## Progressions

- Tricep Kickbacks without weights will be easier for less fit participants or those with a wrist injury (see exercise 15, page 139).
- Start with the buttocks on the floor and progressively add resistance to the movement by lifting the buttocks, extending the legs, and performing from a bench, as illustrated above, to move through a greater range of motion.
- Perform the exercise at a slow pace so the muscles have to contract and work for longer.
- Vary the speed of the exercise, for example two slow double time and four normal pace.
- Perform through different ranges of motion, i.e. halfway up and down, all the way up and halfway down, up again and all the way down, all the way up and down.
- Combine with a knee extension to add variation (ensure both legs receive equal work).
- Use a partner to press on the shoulders to add further resistance to the movement. *Note:* partner work needs to be conducted with great care.
- Perform with the feet and arms raised on different benches to add further resistance to the movement.

## Ex 8    Press-ups and hover press

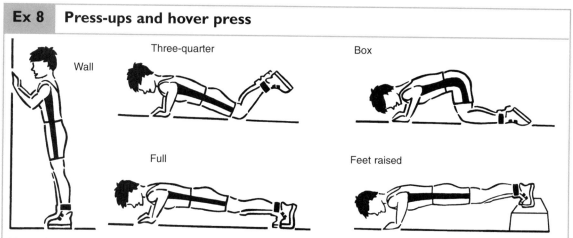

*Note:* the positions illustrated show methods of progressively increasing the resistance to this exercise.

### Purpose

This exercise will work the muscles at the front of the chest and shoulder (the pectorals and anterior deltoids) and the muscles at the back of the upper arm (the triceps).

### Starting position and instructions

Start in one of the five positions illustrated above. Place the hands a shoulder width and a half apart and level with the shoulders, with the fingers facing forwards. Bend and straighten the elbows to lower and lift the body weight up and down. Continue for the desired number of repetitions.

### Teaching points

- Keep the abdominals pulled in tight and the back straight.
- Keep the whole of the spine and neck in line.
- Ensure the elbows fully extend but do not lock.
- Keep the body weight forwards and over the shoulders to maximise the resistance.
- If kneeling in the box or three quarter position take care not to rest on the knee caps.
- Ensure the body lowers and lifts in one smooth movement.

- The chest should touch the floor between the shoulder blades.
- Maintain a right angle (90°) at the elbow joint, keeping the elbow and wrist aligned.

### Progressions

- Perform the exercise at a slow pace so that the muscles have to contract and work for longer.
- Build up to higher repetitions in each position to increase endurance; when 20 repetitions can be achieved, try a harder position.
- Vary the speed of the exercise, for example two slow double time and four normal pace.
- Combine a Leg Curl in between full Press-ups to add variety for stronger participants.
- Adding a clap will make the movement more explosive.
- As a variation, perform with the hands shoulder width apart (narrow). Ensure the elbows move backwards rather than out-wards to maintain the correct elbow and wrist alignment.

To Hover:
Hold down in lower position.
Take care not to hold breath.

| Ex 9 | Back extensions |
|---|---|

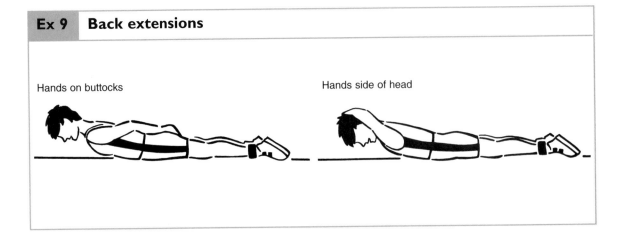

Hands on buttocks

Hands side of head

## Purpose

This exercise will work the muscles that run along the length of the spine (the erector spinae).

## Starting position and instructions

Lie face down on the floor. Place the hands either at the side of the head or on the buttocks, as illustrated above. Pull the abdominals in tight to fix the spine. Raise and lower the chest, keeping the movement controlled at all times.

## Teaching points

- Keep the neck in line with the rest of the spine.
- Keep the abdominals pulled in tight and take care not to hollow the back.
- Lift to a comfortable height.
- Control the movement and breathe comfortably throughout.

## Progressions

- To make the exercise easier, perform with the hands resting on the floor in front of the body and use them to support some of the body weight. Ensure that the arms are not used to push the body up from the floor.
- Progressively add resistance by placing the hands on the buttocks, at the side of the head, and extending the arms (Superman) in line with the rest of the spine.
- Perform the exercise at a slow pace so that the muscle has to contract for a longer period of time.
- Combine with Prone Flyes (exercise 10) to add variety for participants with greater motor skills.
- Use core ball.

## Ex 10    Prone flyes

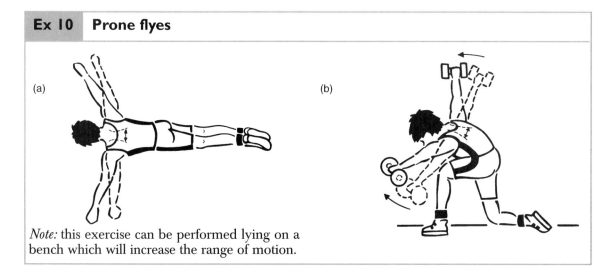

(a)

(b)

*Note:* this exercise can be performed lying on a bench which will increase the range of motion.

### Purpose

This exercise will work the muscles in the middle of the back (the trapezius).

### Starting position and instructions

Start either (a) lying or (b) kneeling in the positions illustrated above. Keep the elbows bent and out to the side of the body, level with shoulders. Raise the arms from the floor using the muscles in the middle of the back. Lower them back to the starting position under control.

### Teaching points

- Raise the arms under control.
- Keep the abdominals pulled in tight and take care not to hollow the back
- Keep the elbows slightly bent throughout the movement.
- Initiate the movement from the middle of the back.
- Take care not to let the arms initiate and dictate the movement; use the arms as resistance.
- If kneeling on one leg take care not to rest on the knee cap and ensure the chest is able to rest comfortably on the thigh.

- If lying, keep the hip bones pressed towards the floor and lift the bellybutton towards the back bone.

### Progressions

- To make the exercise easier, start with the hands on the floor at the side of the buttocks and gently lift the shoulders up from the floor, squeezing the shoulder blades together.
- Perform the exercise at a slow pace so that the muscles have to contract and work for longer.
- Vary the speed of the exercise, for example two slow double time and four normal pace.
- Progress by extending the leverage with the arms out to the side and the elbows bent, and then with the arms out to the side and extended (keep a slight bend in the elbow).
- Add weights to make the exercise harder.
- Combine with back extensions for variety.
- Perform in a kneeling position to increase the range of motion.
- Perform from a step (illustrated in chapter 8) to increase the range of motion.
- Use core ball.

# RESISTANCE EXERCISES USING BARBELLS AND DUMBBELLS

The exercises illustrated in the following pages can be used to design a body sculpt session.

| Ex 1 | Dead lifts |
|---|---|

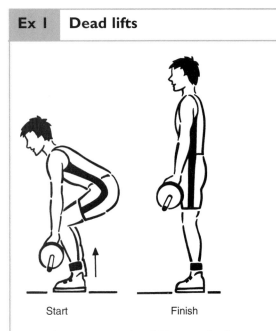

Start          Finish

*Note:* this exercise should be used whenever a weight or object needs to be lifted to the thighs. It allows the weight to be carried by the strength of the thigh muscles and therefore prevents injury to the back when lifting incorrectly

## Purpose

This exercise will work the buttock muscles (the gluteus maximus), the back muscles (the erector spinae), and the muscles at the front of the thighs (the quadriceps).

## Starting position and instructions

Stand and place the toes underneath the barbell, approximately hip width apart. Ensure the body is positioned central to the barbell. Bend at the knees and hips and take an overhand grip of the bar. Lift the bar from the floor by straightening the knees and hips and leading the movement with the shoulders.

## Teaching points

- Ensure that the back is straight and abdominals pulled in.
- Take care not to hollow the back.
- Push the buttocks backwards; avoid letting the knees travel too far in front of the bar.
- The backside should be higher than the knees when bending to reach the bar.
- Look forwards and slightly up.
- Keep the bar close to the body throughout the movement.
- Ensure the body moves to a fully extended position without locking the joints (hip and knee fully straightened and spine extended).

## Progressions

- Perform the exercise without a barbell to get used to the position.
- Start by lifting a light weight and progress to a heavier weight.
- Start at a slow pace so that the muscles have to contract and work for longer.
- Vary the speed of the movements, some very slow (four counts down and four counts up) and some to normal time.
- Combine with a Calf Raise or Upright Row to add variety to the movement. These two variations provide a method for breaking down and introducing the next lift 'clean' into the session.
- Perform with wider grip for persons with limited shoulder mobility.

## Ex 2 Upright rows

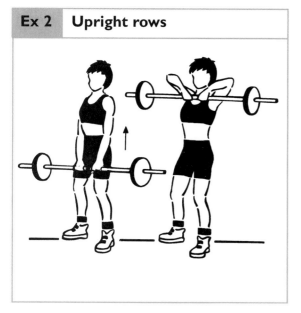

### Purpose

This exercise will work the muscles at the front of the shoulder (anterior deltoids), the front of the upper arm (the biceps and brachialis), and the top of the back (the trapezius).

### Starting position and instructions

Dead lift the barbell to the thighs using an overhand grip. Widen the foot stance to a hip width and a half apart. Narrow the bar grip to double thumb width apart. Keep a firm grip of the bar with the thumbs tucked under. Raise the bar towards the chin, keeping the bar close to the body. Lower the bar under control. Continue for the desired number of repetitions.

### Teaching points

- Keep the bar close to the body.
- Keep the abdominals pulled in tight, and avoid hollowing the lower back on the downward phase.
- Keep the movement controlled.
- Tuck the bottom in and keep the knees unlocked.
- Lead the movement with the elbows, lifting them as high as possible (up to the chin).

### Progressions

- Perform without a weight to rehearse the movement.
- Perform with a light barbell and progressively add resistance.
- Perform at a slow pace so that the muscles have to contract and work for longer.
- Combine with a Dead Lift to perform part of 'The Clean'.

## Ex 3 | Calf raises

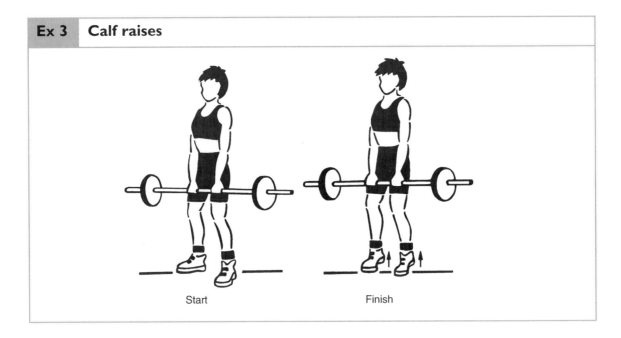

Start                    Finish

## Purpose

This exercise will work the muscles at the back of the lower leg (the gastrocnemius and soleus).

## Starting position and instructions

Start with the feet hip width apart. Dead lift the barbell to the thighs using an overhand grip. Keep the bar still. Rise on to the balls of the feet, lifting the heels from the floor. Lower down under control. Continue for the desired number of repetitions.

## Teaching points

- Keep the bar still and close to the body.
- Keep the abdominals pulled in tight and the back straight.
- Keep the knee joints unlocked.
- Press on to the ball of the foot with the weight central, taking care not to roll the ankles outwards.
- Keep the movement smooth and controlled.

## Progressions

- Perform without a weight to rehearse the movement.
- Perform with a lighter barbell and progressively add resistance.
- Perform at a slow pace so that the muscles have to contract and work for longer.
- Perform with dumbbells to add variety.
- Combine with a Dead Lift to perform part of 'The Clean'.
- Perform with an Upright Row to increase motor skills and rehearse as part of The Clean.

## Ex 4　Dumbbell lunges

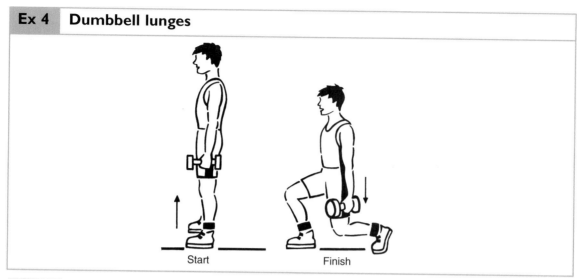

Start　　　　　　　　Finish

### Purpose

This exercise will work the buttock muscles (gluteus maximus) and the muscles at the front of the thighs (quadriceps).

### Starting position and instructions

Stand with the feet hip width apart with dumbbells placed each side of the feet. Dead lift the dumbbells to the thighs. Check that the feet are positioned comfortably with the toes facing forwards. Take a large step forwards and bend the knee to lower the body weight downwards. Ensure both knees are positioned at right angles (90°). Push through the thigh to lift the body back to standing position. Perform either by alternating legs or repeating the movement on the same leg. Dead lift the dumbbells to the floor on completion of the exercise.

### Teaching points

- Ensure the front knee does not overshoot the toe.
- Step forwards and sink the body down centrally rather than diving forwards into the movement.
- Keep the abdominals pulled in tight and the chest lifted.
- Ensure the knee does not roll inwards.
- Bend the back knee towards the floor, but ensure the knee cap does not crash against the floor.
- Look straight ahead and slightly down.
- Drive through the thigh to return the body to an upright position.
- Keep a relaxed grip on the dumbbells, and keep the shoulders relaxed and pressed down.

### Progressions

- Perform without a weight to rehearse the movement and to familiarise participants with the balance required.
- Perform through a small range of motion initially.
- Start the exercise at a slow pace so that the muscles have to contract and work for longer.
- Start with light dumbbells and progressively add weight.
- Vary the speed of the exercise, for example two slow double time and four normal pace.
- Alternating legs will be slightly easier; repeating a number of repetitions on the same leg will require greater muscular endurance.

| Ex 5 | **Barbell curls** |
|---|---|

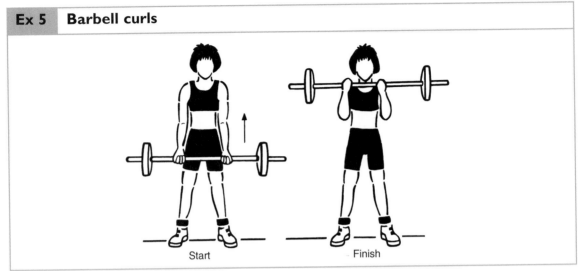

Start          Finish

## Purpose

This exercise will work the muscles at the front of the upper arm (the biceps and brachialis).

## Starting position and instructions

Stand with the feet hip width apart. Dead lift the barbell to the thighs using an underhand grip. Widen the foot stance to a shoulder width and a half apart, and unlock the knees. Narrow the hand grip of the barbell to a shoulder width apart. Fix the elbows close to the side of the body. Keep the body lifted and buttocks tucked in. Curl the bar in an arc-like motion towards the chest. Lower the bar to the thighs, fully extending, but not locking, the elbows.

## Teaching points

- Raise the bar under control.
- Keep the abdominals pulled in tight taking care not to hollow or swing the back.
- Keep the wrists fixed and straight.

- Keep the elbows and upper arms close to the body.
- The lower arms should be the only body parts moving.
- Avoid locking the elbows when the bar lowers and the arms fully extend.

## Progressions

- Perform without a bar (or a light bar) to rehearse the skills.
- Progressively add more weight to the movement.
- Perform at a slow pace so that the muscles have to contract and work for longer.
- Vary the speed of the exercise, for example two slow double time and four normal pace.
- Perform through different ranges of motion, i.e. halfway up and down, all the way up and halfway down, up again and all the way down, all the way up and down.
- Perform with dumbbells to add variety.
- Use dumbbells and core ball.

## Ex 6  Dumbbell lateral raises

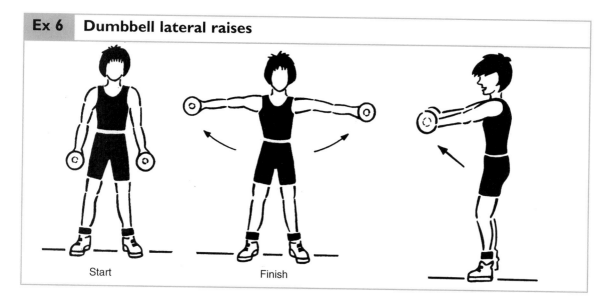

Start                          Finish

## Purpose

This exercise will work the shoulder muscles (the deltoids).

## Starting position and instructions

Stand with the feet hip width apart. Dead lift the dumbbells to the thighs. Widen the foot stance to a hip width and a half apart. Position the dumbbells at the side of the thighs. Raise the dumbbells out to the side of the body to shoulder height. Lower the dumbbells under control.

## Teaching points

- Lead the movement with the knuckles and keep the wrists fixed.
- Keep the elbows slightly bent throughout the movement.
- Keep the abdominals pulled in tight and the bottom tucked in.
- Rotate the dumbbells as they are lifted so that the thumbs tilt forwards.
- Avoid any excess movement at the top of the back.
- Keep the movement controlled and smooth.

## Progressions

- Perform without weights to rehearse the movement.
- Perform the exercise at a slow pace so that the muscles have to contract and work for longer.
- Vary the speed of the exercise: use some slow time and some normal time.
- Combine with a Dumbbell Lunge to challenge motor skills.
- Perform with a travelling Side Squat as illustrated in chapter 5.
- Perform seated on core ball.

# CLEAN-BASED LIFTS

| Ex 7 | The clean |
|------|-----------|

Step one     Step two     Step three     Step four     Step five

*Safety note:* this is an extremely complex lift. This exercise needs to be supervised and instructed by a qualified resistance training teacher. It should not be performed unsupervised by individuals who are inexperienced at working with weights. It is explained and illustrated in this book purely to show readers an appropriate method for lifting a weight to the shoulders in preparation to push press the bar behind the neck. It will need to be performed to move the barbell into position for the Back Squat and behind Neck Press. It is not intended to be performed as a specific exercise.

## Purpose

This exercise works many of the major muscles: the buttock muscles (the gluteus maximus), the back muscles (the erector spinae), the muscles at the front of the thighs (the quadriceps), the calf muscles (the gastrocnemius and soleus), the shoulder muscles (the deltoids), the middle and upper back muscles (the trapezius), and the muscles at the front of the upper arm (the biceps).

## Starting position and instructions

**Step one**: Dead lift the bar to the thighs (see 'Teaching points' for Dead Lift).
**Step two**: Upright row the bar and calf raise (see 'Teaching points' for Upright Row and Calf Raise).
**Step three**: Receive – bring the elbows forwards and under the bar so that the bar rests under the shoulders, at the same time lowering the heels and bending the knees to cushion the weight.

Stand up straight. Note: the bar should remain in the same position.
**Step four**: Return – bring the elbows back around to Upright Row position. *Note*: keep the bar close to the body and the elbows high. Lower the bar to the thighs.
**Step five**: Reverse dead lift the bar to the floor (*see* 'Teaching points' for Dead Lift).

## Teaching points

- Keep the back straight.
- Keep the abdominals pulled in throughout the movement.

## Progressions

- Perform the exercise without a barbell to get used to the movement.
- Perform the exercise slowly and in separate stages to get used to each step.
- Aim to perform as a smooth and fluid movement.

| Ex 8 | Back squats |
|---|---|

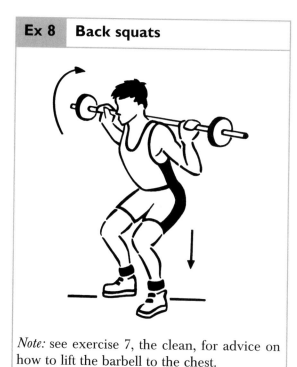

*Note:* see exercise 7, the clean, for advice on how to lift the barbell to the chest.

## Purpose

This exercise will work the buttock muscles (the gluteus maximus) and the muscles at the front of the thighs (the quadriceps).

## Starting position and instructions

Clean the barbell to the 'receive' position. Push press the bar over the head and rest it at the back of the shoulders (bend the knees and push through the thighs to assist movement of the bar). Widen the bar grip to a comfortable position. Ensure the feet are placed comfortably hip width apart. Bend the knees and lower the body downwards. Return to an upright position to complete the lift. Continue for the desired number of repetitions. To return the bar push press the bar back over the head and rest it at the front of the chest and shoulders, and return as for The Clean.

## Teaching points

- Look forwards throughout the movement.
- Keep the knees travelling in line with the feet.
- Do not let the bottom drop below the knees when squatting downwards: this will place a lot of stress on the knee joints.
- Keep the back straight.
- Squat down so that the bar moves in a straight and vertical line.
- When straightening the knees do not lock them.
- Fully extend the hips and knees.

## Progressions

- Perform without a weight to rehearse the movement.
- Perform at a slow pace so that the muscles have to contract and work for longer.
- Perform initially through a small range of motion.
- Progressively add weight to the barbell to increase resistance.

## Ex 9 — Behind or front neck presses/shoulder presses

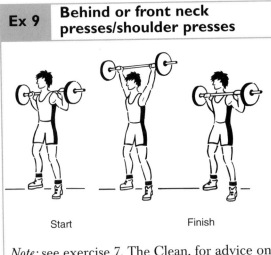

Start           Finish

*Note:* see exercise 7, The Clean, for advice on how to lift the barbell to the chest.

### Purpose

This exercise will work the shoulder muscles (the deltoids), the muscles of the upper back (trapezius), and the muscles at the back of the upper arms (the triceps).

### Starting position and instructions

Clean the barbell to the receive position. Push press the bar over the head and rest at the back of the shoulders. Widen the foot stance to a hip width and a half apart to assist balance. Widen the grip of the bar to a shoulder width and a half apart. Press the bar upwards. Lower the bar down under control. Continue for the desired number of repetitions. Do not allow the bar to rest on the shoulders in between lifts, keep a constant muscle tension. To return the bar, narrow the grip, push press the bar over the head to rest on the front of the chest/shoulders and return as for The Clean.

### Teaching points

- Keep the back straight, abdominals pulled in and bottom tucked under.
- Keep the knuckles facing up and the wrists fixed.
- Take care not to hollow the back or lock the elbows.
- Keep the knees slightly bent throughout the movement.
- Keep a smooth and comfortable movement.

### Progressions

- Perform without a weight to rehearse the movement.
- Add weight progressively to challenge the muscles.
- Perform the exercise at a slower pace so that the muscles have to contract and work for longer.
- Vary the speed of the exercise: two slow counts up and down (double time) and four normal counts up and down.
- Can press from front of body for persons with limited shoulder mobility.

# BENCH LIFTS

In a weight training environment all bench lifts should be performed using a spotter, particularly when they are performed by inexperienced participants, and/or when heavier weights are being used. Because this book is about exercise to music, *it is assumed that the weights being lifted will not be maximal* and will only be introduced to participants who have some training experience. Appropriate methods of moving the bar into position for bench lifts that are used within an ETM class are outlined in table 9.4.

| Table 9.4 | Positioning the bar for bench lifts in a body sculpt session |
|---|---|
| If using light weights with participants who have a reasonable level of experience, it is appropriate to roll the barbell or dumbbells into position and this can be achieved in the following ways. | |
| *Barbell* | • Dead lift the bar to the thighs and sit down on the bench with the bar resting on the thighs.<br>• Lie flat on the bench and roll the body towards the chest. Take the appropriate grip of the bar and perform the lift.<br>• Return the bar using the same principles (roll back, stand up and return dead lift). |
| *Dumbbells* | • Dead lift the dumbbells to the thighs and sit down on the bench with the dumbbells resting on the thighs.<br>• Lie flat on the bench and lift alternate dumbells to the chest.<br>• Return the dumbbells using the same principles (place back, sit up, stand up and return dead lift). |

| Ex 10 | **Bench presses** |
|---|---|

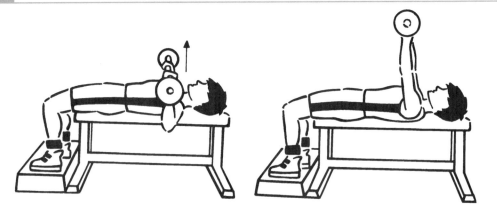

*Note:* if the back hollows, rest the feet on a step. This provides better balance and is generally more secure and safer than placing the feet on the bench.

## Purpose

This exercise will work the muscles at the front of the chest (the pectorals), the muscles at the front of the shoulders (the anterior deltoids), and the muscles at the back of the upper arms (the triceps).

## Starting position and instructions

Move the bar into position using the technique explained in table 9.4. Position the hands on the bar a shoulder width and half apart. Push the bar straight up to the ceiling. Lower the bar back to the chest, controlling the movement. Perform the desired number of repetitions. To return the bar, use the technique explained in table 9.4.

## Teaching points

- Keep the knuckles facing upwards and the wrists fixed.
- Keep the abdominals pulled in tight taking care not to hollow the back (see note above).

- Move the bar in a straight line and level with the chest.
- Extend the arms fully, but do not lock the elbows.
- Keep the elbows and wrists in line and vertical as the bar lowers.
- Keep the movement smooth and controlled.

## Progressions

- Perform without a weight to rehearse the movement.
- Perform the exercise at a slow pace so the muscles have to contract and work for longer.
- Vary the speed of the exercise, performing some repetitions at slow time and some at normal pace.
- Perform through different ranges of motion (lower range, upper range, full range).
- Progressively add greater resistance to the movement by lifting a heavier weight.

## Ex 11    Bent arm pullovers

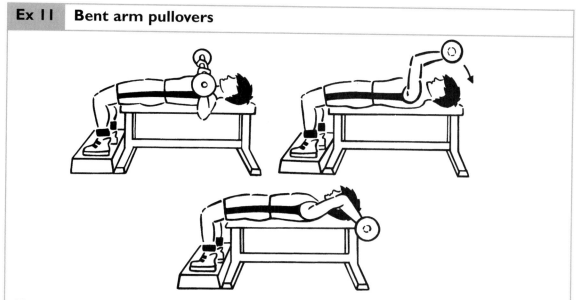

*Note:* if the back hollows, rest the feet on a step. This provides better balance and is generally more secure and safer than placing the feet on the bench.

### Purpose

This exercise will work the muscles at the front of the chest (the pectorals) and the muscles at the side of the back (the latissimus dorsi).

### Starting position and instructions

Get the bar into position using the technique explained in table 9.4. Take a shoulder width, narrow grip of the bar. Press the bar to the ceiling and lower it down so that the elbows are pressed into the sides of the body and the wrists (and bar) are in line with the elbows. Keep this 90° angle at the elbow throughout the movement. Take the bar over the head, keeping the elbows fixed and in line with the wrists, and lower the bar towards the floor at the back of the bench. Return by reversing the movement and leading with the elbows to bring the bar back towards the chest. Perform the desired number of repetitions. To return the bar use the technique explained in table 9.4.

### Teaching points

- Move the bar with controlled movements.
- Keep the abdominals pulled in tight and take care not to hollow the back, especially as the bar moves over the head and towards the floor.
- Keep the elbows bent and pressed inwards (not splaying out) throughout the movement.
- Breathe in a controlled manner throughout the exercise.

### Progressions

- Perform without a weight so that the correct alignment can be rehearsed.
- Progressively add weight to the movement by lifting a heavier barbell.
- Perform the exercise at a slow pace so that the muscles have to contract and work for longer.

## Ex 12　Lying tricep extensions

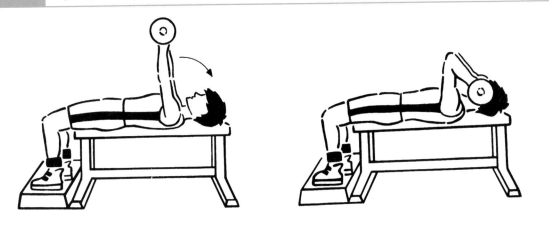

*Note:* if the back hollows, rest the feet on a step. This provides better balance and is generally more secure and safer than placing the feet on the bench.

### Purpose

This exercise will work the muscles at the back of the upper arms (the triceps).

### Starting position and instructions

Get the bar into position, using the technique explained in table 9.4. Take a shoulder width, narrow grip of the bar. Press the bar to the ceiling, keeping it level with the chest. Keep the upper arms fixed in this position. Bend the lower arms so that the barbell moves downwards towards the bridge of the nose. Return the barbell back towards the ceiling. Perform the desired number of repetitions. Return the bar using the technique explained in table 9.4.

### Teaching points

- Keep the wrists and elbows fixed throughout the movement.
- Keep the abdominals pulled in tight and take care not to hollow the back.
- Move the bar with controlled movements.
- Straighten the arms fully, but without locking the elbows.

### Progressions

- Perform the exercise without a weight to rehearse the movement.
- Perform the exercise at a slow pace so that the muscles have to contract and work for longer.
- Vary the speed by performing some slow and extra slow counts, and some normal pace counts.
- For advanced and more flexible participants, take the bar down over the head. This will provide a greater range of motion and target the longer head of the tricep muscle.

| Ex 13 | Lying dumbbell flyes |

*Note:* if the back hollows, rest the feet on a step. This provides better balance and is generally more secure and safer than placing the feet on the bench.

## Purpose

This exercise will work the chest muscles (pectorals).

## Starting position and instructions

Move the dumbbells into position by using the technique explained in table 9.4. Press the dumbbells to the ceiling so they are level with the chest, with the palms facing inwards. Keep the elbows unlocked and the arms fixed in this position. Lower the dumbbells out to each side of the body so they are parallel to the floor. Return the dumbbells back towards the body. Perform the desired number of repetitions. Return the bar using the technique explained in table 9.4.

## Teaching points

- Move the dumbbells with control.
- Keep the abdominals pulled in tight and take care not to hollow the back.
- Keep the wrists, elbows and shoulders in line throughout the movement.
- Keep the wrists fixed and the elbows unlocked.

## Progressions

- Perform the exercise without weights to rehearse the movement.
- Perform at a slow pace so that the muscles have to contract and work for longer.
- Vary the speed of the exercise by performing some slow double time repetitions and some normal pace repetitions.
- Progressively add weight to increase the resistance being lifted.
- This exercise can be performed on an incline or decline to concentrate on a different area of the muscle.
- Perform on core ball.

## Ex 14 Single arm rows

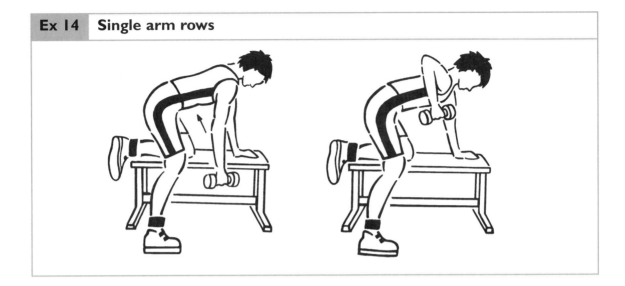

### Purpose

This exercise will work the muscles at the back (the latissimus dorsi) and the muscles at the front of the upper arms (the biceps).

### Starting position and instructions

Position the dumbbell at the side of the bench. Place one knee and one hand on the bench with the other foot level with the knee and forming a triangular base of support. Keep the weight-bearing knee slightly bent. Bend the knee further and extend the arm to reach for the dumbbell. Straighten the leg to lift the dumbbell into position. Draw the dumbbell towards the armpit, keeping the dumbbell close to the body. Lower the dumbbell back down so that the arm is extended. Repeat for the desired number of repetitions. Perform using the other arm.

### Teaching points

- Keep the back straight and look forwards throughout the movement.
- Keep the abdominals pulled in tight.
- Ensure the elbow does not lock as the dumbbell lowers back down.
- Take care not to twist the back or shoulders.
- Keep the shoulders square.

### Progressions

- Perform without the dumbbell to rehearse the movement.
- Perform the exercise at a slow pace.
- Vary the pace, for example two slow double time lifts and four normal pace lifts.
- Combine with exercise 15, Triceps Kickbacks, to add variety for participants with greater motor skills.

| Ex 15 | Triceps kickbacks |

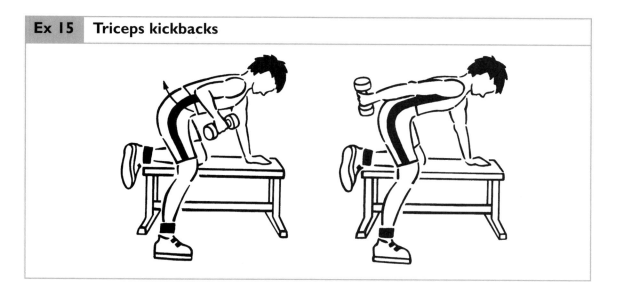

## Purpose

This exercise will work the muscles at the back of the upper arm (the triceps).

## Starting position and instructions

Position the dumbbell at the side of the bench. Place one knee and one hand on the bench with the foot level with the other knee and forming a triangular base of support. Keep the weight-bearing knee slightly bent. Bend the knee further and extend the arm to reach for the dumbbell. Straighten the leg to lift the dumbbell into position. Draw the dumbbell upwards so that the upper arm is pressed into the side of the body. Hold this position. Extend the elbow backwards, keeping the upper arm fixed and the dumbbell close to the body. Return by bringing the dumbbell back to the first position. Repeat for the desired number of repetitions. Perform using the other arm.

## Teaching points

- Move the dumbbell with control and do not allow the weight to swing.
- Keep the abdominals pulled in tight and take care not to twist or hollow the back.
- Extend the elbow fully without locking or hyperextending the joint.
- Keep the shoulders square throughout the movement.

## Progressions

- Perform the exercise without the dumbbell, or use a light weight to rehearse the technique.
- Perform at a slow pace so that the muscles have to contract and work for longer.
- Vary the speed of the exercise by combining slow time and normal time repetitions.
- Combine with Single Arm Rows (exercise 14) to add variety.

## Ex 16 | Overhead tricep press

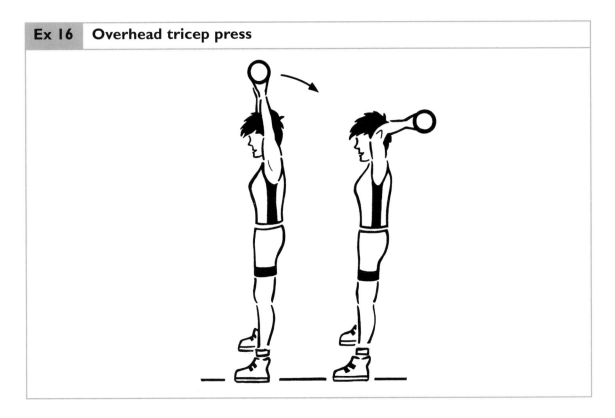

## Purpose

This exercise will work the muscles at the back of the upper arm (triceps)

## Instructions

Standing feet hip width apart or stagger foot stance so that one foot is in front of the other. Hold a dumbbell with both hands.
Raise the dumbbell overhead.
Lower the dumbbell behind the head, bending at elbows.
Straighten the arms to return the dumbbell over head.

## Teaching points

• Abdominals pulled in
• Chest lifted and shoulders relaxed.
• Fully bend and straighten arms without locking elbows.
• Keep elbows close to head.

## Adaptation

• Perform seated on bench or swiss ball.
• Use single arm to hold dumbbell
• Vary speed, repetitions and resistance to accommodate individuals
• Perform tricep kick backs or dips as an alternative.

## Ex 17 Bent over row

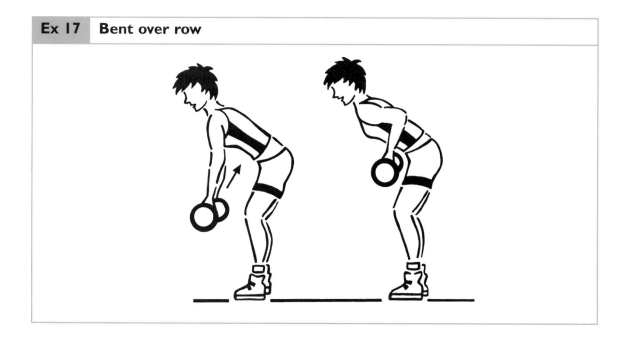

### Purpose

This exercise will work the muscles at the side of the back (latissimus dorsi) and the front of the upper arms (biceps)

### Instructions

Feet hip width apart.
Bend forward from the hip 45 degrees
Holding the bar bell towards the floor (arms straight) shoulder width apart.
Pull the barbell to the upper abdomen.
Lower under control.

### Teaching points

- Maintain a neutral pelvic alignment and pull abdominals in
- Shoulders relaxed and down
- Lengthen the neck
- Elbows close to body
- Knees slightly bent throughout.
- Keep the spine long.
- Elbows unlocked as arm straightens.

### Adaptation

- Take a wider grip (shoulder width and half apart and row the bar to upper abdominals squeezing the shoulder blades back, elbows out to side) to work trapezius.
- Vary speed, repetitions, resistance to accommodate different abilities.
- Use exercise band instead of free weight.
- Perform single arm row as alternative.

| Table 9.5 | Example of partial lesson plan for an introductory body sculpt session |
|---|---|
| **Component and exercise** | **Repetitions** |
| Warm-up (mobility, pulse-raising, prep stretch) *See chapter 5 for appropriate exercises.* | Without resistance |
| Re-warmer | Without resistance for beginners; light resistance for intermediate/advanced |
| • Dead Lift | 12–15 reps |
| • Calf Raise | 12–15 reps |
| • Upright Row | 12–15 reps |
| Repeat | |
| • Dumbbell Lunge | 12–15 reps |
| • Lateral Raise | 12–15 reps |
| Main workout with weights | Select appropriate resistance |
| • Combined Dead Lift/Calf Raise/Upright Row  Teach receive and return phases of The Clean  Teach push press | 10–12 reps |
| • Repeat Dead Lift/Calf Raise/Upright Row combo  Receive and push press | 10–12 reps |
| • Back Squat | 12–15 reps |
| • Behind Neck Press | 8–10 reps |
| Repeat | |
| Return bar to floor | |
| Dead Lift with underhand grip | |
| • Barbell Curl | 12–15 reps |
| Main workout with bench lifts | Select appropriate resistance |
| • Single Arm Row | 15 reps |
| • Tricep Extension | 10 reps |
| Repeat on the other arm | |
| Repeat again on both arms | |
| Cool-down (pulse-lowering stretch, re-mobilise) *See chapter 6 for appropriate exercises.* | It may be necessary to re-warm the muscles before stretching, rather than pulse-lowering. |

*Note:* appropriate exercises for the abdominal and trapezius muscles will need to be included in the main workout to achieve a more balanced whole body approach (*see* resistance exercises 1 (page 126), 2 (page 127), 3 (page 128) and 10 (page 135)).

| Table 9.6 | General mobility and pulse raising for body conditioning class – (Mixed ability) | | |
|---|---|---|---|
| **Timing** | **Exercise Description and Purpose** | **Alternative For less skilled** | **Progression For more skilled** |
| 8 Rt × 1 8 Lt × 1 4 – 4 × 2 2 – 2 × 4 1 – 1 × 8 | Toe taps Pick up beat of music *Slight ankle mobility* | 8 counts and 4 counts only | Add hip wiggle |
| 1 × 16 | Step tap Pick up beat of music *Gentle pulse raising* | | Bend deeper |
| 1 × 16 | Step tap and shoulder lifts Mobilise shoulders | Isolate shoulder lifts | |
| 1 × 16 | Step tap and shoulder rolls *Mobilise shoulders* | Isolate shoulder rolls | |
| 1 × 16 | Step tap and reach arms in front *Pulse raising and shoulder mobility* | Step tap without reach | |
| 1 × 16 | Step tap and reach arms over head | Keep arms to front | |
| 4 × 16 | Leg curls with arm pull backs 4 face front 4 turning – 90 degrees each turn (so full turn achieved) *Knee mobility and pulse raise* repeat × 4 times through | Leg curls, no turn. Decrease reps | Bend deeper |
| | Can repeat shoulder mobility if necessary | | |
| 4 × 16 | Side step right × 2 Side step left × 2 Arms raise to side *Pulse raise* Repeat | Leave out arms | Bend deeper Vary arm line Add a jump to the side step Grapevine |
| 2 × 16 | Step and knee lifts with arm pull downs *Hip mobility and pulse raise* | Leave out arms Bicep curl arms | Travel forward × 4 Static × 4 Travel back × 4 Static × 4 Can add full turn on static lifts. 90 degree turn on each step |
| | Can repeat leg curls, side steps and knee lifts if necessary | | |
| 2 × 16 | Walk forward and back | Smaller strides | Walk to diagonals |
| | Back lunges into calf stretch | | |

| Table 9.7 | General preparatory (warm up) stretching for body conditioning class ( Mixed ability) | | |
|---|---|---|---|
| **Timing** | **Exercise Description and Purpose** | **Alternative For less skilled** | **Progression For more skilled** |
| 1 × 32 | A. Walk forward (right leg lead) and back | Smaller stride | Longer stride |
| 1 × 16 10 secs | B. Back lunges (right leg lead) Into static *calf stretch* right | Smaller lunge | Combine with pectoral stretch |
| 10 secs | Static quad stretch right | Hold wall for balance | Can bend and straighten support knee whilst stretching |
| 10 secs | Static *hamstring stretch* right | Smaller bend at hip | Lift buttock higher on stretching leg |
| 1 × 16 | Wide squats | Shallow bend | Deeper bend |
| 1 × 16 | Side twists *Spine mobility* | | |
| 1 × 16 | Side bends *Spine mobility* | | |
| 1 × 16 10 secs | Wide squats Into double adductor stretch | Single leg adductor stretch | Single leg adductor stretch with oblique stretch |
| 1 × 32 1 × 16 | Repeat A and B (left leg lead) | | Combine calf stretch with trapezius stretch |
| 10 secs × 3 | Repeat stretches left leg | | |
| 1 × 32 | Step tap | Isolate stretches without leg movement | Triceps only if other stretches combined with lower body stretches. |
| 10 secs 10 secs 10 secs | *Stretch triceps* R and L *Stretch pectorals* *Stretch trapezius* | | |
| 1 × 16 | C. Walk forwards and backwards Pulse raising | | |
| 1 × 16 | D. Side lunges with lateral raise Pulse raising | Leave out arms | Deeper bend |
| 1 × 32 | Repeat C and D above | | |

*NB*: For specific progressions and adaptations for each stretch position refer to chapter 5.

| Table 9.8 | Standing MSE for body conditioning class (Mixed ability) | | |
|---|---|---|---|
| **Reps, Speed & Stick diagram** | **Exercise Description and Purpose** | **Alternative (For less fit)** | **Progression (For more advanced)** |
| 1-1 × 32 | A. Standing<br>Step left and Side leg raise right combine with dumbbell lateral raise<br>*Abductors and Deltoids* | 1 × 16 reps<br>Isolate legs and then arms | Increase dumbbell weight |
| 1-1 × 32 | B. Standing _ turn to left step left forward and gluteal raise right combine with bicep curls<br>*Gluteus Maximus and Biceps* | 1 × 16 reps<br>Isolate legs and then arms | Increase dumbbell weight |
| 1-1 × 16 | C. March and face front | | |
| 1-1 × 16<br>2-2 × 8<br>1-3 × 4<br>3-1 × 4 | D. Wide Squats<br>*Quads, Gluteals, Hamstrings* | 1-1 × 16<br>2-2 × 8<br>no weights | Extra sets:<br>1-7 × 2<br>7-1 × 2<br>Increase dumbbell weight |
| | Repeat A and B with right leg tap and left leg raise | | |
| 1-1 × 16<br>2-2 × 8<br>1-3 × 4<br>3-1 × 4 | E. Narrow squats<br>*Quads, Gluteals, Hamstrings* | 1-1 × 16<br>2-2 × 8<br>no weights | Extra sets:<br>1-7 × 2<br>7-1 × 2<br>Increase dumbbell weight |
| 2-2 × 16 | F. Upright row<br>*Anterior Deltoid, Biceps, upper trapezius.* | 1 × 12 | Increase resistance |
| 2-2 × 16 | G. Shoulder press<br>*Deltoids, Triceps, upper Trapezius* | 1 × 12 | Increase resistance |
| | Repeat F and G to superset | No repeat or rest between sets | |
| 2-2 × 16 | H. Bicep curl<br>*Biceps* | 1 × 12 | Increase resistance |
| 2-2 × 16 | I. Tricep press<br>*Triceps* | 1 × 12 | Increase resistance |
| | Repeat H and I to superset | No repeat or rest between sets | |

| Table 9.9 | Floor based MSE for body conditioning class (Mixed ability) | | |
|---|---|---|---|
| **Reps, Speed & Stick diagram** | **Exercise Description and Purpose** | **Alternative (For less fit)** | **Progression (For more advanced)** |
| 1-1 × 20 | Supine crook lying (on back with knees bent)<br>A. Curl up<br>*Rectus abdominus* | 1 × 12-16 rest before next exercise | 1-1 × 8<br>2-2 × 8<br>3-1 × 4<br>1-3 × 4 |
| 1-1 × 20 | Supine crook lying<br>B. Twisting sit up<br>*Obliques* | 1 × 12-16 rest before next exercise | Add bicycle legs |
| 1-1 × 20 | Supine lying with knees raised<br>C. Reverse curls<br>*Rectus abdominus* | 1 × 12-16 | |
| 1-1 × 24 | Left side lying<br>D. Side leg raise<br>*Abductors* | 1 × 20 | 2-2 × 16<br>1-1 × 8 |
| 1-1 × 24 | Left side lying<br>E. Inner thigh raises<br>Adductors | 1 × 20 | 2-2 × 16<br>1-1 × 8 |
| | Repeat A, B and C | | |
| | Right side lying<br>Repeat D and E | | |
| 2-2 × 16<br>1-1 × 8 | F. _ press ups<br>Pectorals, Triceps, Anterior Deltoid | Box press up<br>1-1 × 12/16 | Replace single count sets with<br>3-1 × 4<br>1-3 × 4<br>or full press ups |
| 1-1 × 16 | Prone lying (on front)<br>G. Back extensions – hands side of head<br>*Erector Spinae* | 1 × 12 hands on lower back | 1 × 20 or combine with prone flye |
| 1-1 × 16 | Prone lying<br>H. Prone flyes<br>*Middle Trapezius and Rhomboids* | 1 × 12 | Use dumbbells if isolating |
| | Repeat F, G and H | | |
| 1-1 × 24 | Prone kneeling, right leg raised<br>I. Gluteal raise<br>*Gluteus maximus* | Lying gluteal raises<br><br>1 × 16 | Add extra set:<br>1 × 16 top range pulse |
| | Repeat I with left leg | | |
| | Prone lying: Front thigh and abdominal stretch | | |

*NB*: any progressions and adaptations suggested are guidelines. They are not golden rules. Teachers should observe their class and adapt as appropriate.

| Table 9.10 | Post workout stretch – for body conditioning class (Mixed ability) | | |
|---|---|---|---|
| **Length of hold & Stick diagram** | **Exercise Description and Purpose** | **Alternative position & stick diagram** | **Progression and adaptation** |
| 30 secs develop R & L | Supine lying – hamstrings | Seated hamstrings | P – ease leg straighter<br><br>A – Hold a towel around leg |
| 15 secs maintain R & L | Supine lying – gluteal stretch | Seated gluteal stretch | P – ease leg closer<br>A – Keep leg on floor |
| 15 secs maintain R & L | Supine lying – oblique stretch | Seated oblique stretch | P – take legs closer to floor, hold longer<br>A – Only a small bend |
| 30 seconds | Seated adductor stretch | Seated straddle/ wide leg position | P – ease knees down further<br>A – Hands on floor behind back to assist upright sitting position. |
| 10 – 15 secs maintain R & L | Seated tricep stretch | Take arm across the front of the body (stretches posterior deltoid and little tricep) | P – use other arm behind back & link hands to increase stretch<br>A – press from front |
| 15 secs maintain | Seated pectoral stretch | Standing if seated position uncomfortable for back | P- raise arms slightly higher<br>A – place hands on floor behind back |
| 10 secs maintain | Seated trapezius stretch | Standing if seated position uncomfortable for back | P – wrap arms around body and drop head forward<br>A – small round of upper back. |
| 15 secs | Standing calf stretch | Seated with legs out straight. Place right heel on top of left foot and use heel to draw toes of lower leg towards knee | P – use wall to lean further into stretch<br>A – use wall for balance |

*NB*: Quads and rectus abdominus stretched at end of floor MSE work.

# DESIGNING A CIRCUIT TRAINING PROGRAMME

10

## Why use circuit training?

Circuit training can provide an effective alternative to the traditional ETM programme. Exercises to train all the components of fitness can still be included and the circuit theme will add variety to the programme for regular exercisers. This may attract interest from new participants, particularly male participants, or individuals who are less keen on what they perceive to be dance-type activities.

## How should a circuit training session be structured?

As with all programmes the session should be preceded by an appropriate warm-up and concluded with an appropriate cool-down. The main workout should comprise a range of exercises designed in a circuit training format; a range of different formats are illustrated in figures 10.1 to 10.5. An outline of the necessary session structure is provided in table 10.1.

## What type of exercises are appropriate to use in a circuit training session?

If the aim of the circuit is to improve purely cardio-vascular fitness, all of the exercises illustrated at the end of chapters 7 and 8 will be appropriate. If the aim of the circuit is to improve muscular strength and endurance, the exercises illustrated at the end of chapter 9 will

be appropriate. If a combined cardio-vascular fitness and muscular strength and endurance workout is the aim, then the exercises in all of the aforementioned chapters are appropriate.

When using a combined approach, it is wise to alternate muscular strength and endurance exercises with cardio-vascular exercises. This should ensure that the intensity of activities is maintained for an appropriate frequency to improve cardio-vascular fitness. This approach is advisable because many of the muscular strength and endurance activities illustrated will not be effective in maintaining the necessary intensity for effective cardio-vascular training; they may lower the intensity too much if performed consecutively in the same circuit.

An alternative approach is to perform two specific circuits: the first circuit consisting of cardio-vascular exercises, and the second consisting of muscular strength and endurance exercises. If two main circuits are used, the intensity of the cardio-vascular circuit will need to be reduced slightly before going on to the muscular strength and endurance circuit. An appropriate session structure to follow for this approach is outlined in table 7.1, page 83.

| Table 10.1 | The structure of a circuit training session |
|---|---|
| *Warm-up* | • Mobility and pulse-raising exercises.<br>• Preparatory stretches.<br>• Re-warm (increasing intensity to the level of the circuit). |
| *Main workout – circuit training component (three approaches)* | 1 Specific toning exercises targeting all major muscle groups to achieve a balanced whole body approach and improve muscular strength and endurance.<br>2 A range of specific exercises to target cardio-vascular fitness.<br>3 A combination of both types of exercises to improve both muscular and cardio-vascular components of fitness. |
| *Cool-down* | • Cooling-down, pulse-lowering exercises (lowering intensity from the level of the circuit).<br>• Post-workout stretches (maintenance and developmental).<br>• Relaxation (optional).<br>• Re-mobilise. |

*Note:* the intensity and selection of exercises included in the re-warmer and cool-down will need to correspond to the intensity of the main workout. If the intensity of the main workout is high and includes a number of energetic cardio-vascular movements, then the intensity of all these components will need to be built up and built down respectively.

## How can the circuit be controlled?

Teachers who are dealing with groups of participants will need to plan carefully to ensure adequate control is achieved. Participants will need to be introduced to the stations; if they are not, they may be unsure of how to perform the exercises correctly. Some teachers introduce stations after the re-warmer, however this approach often lowers the intensity unless participants are kept sufficiently active while the exercises are being demonstrated and

explained. A more appropriate method of introducing the exercise stations is to perform each exercise at a lower intensity throughout the warm-up component. This will assist with a progressive rise in intensity and will maintain interest and improve the continuity and flow of the session.

Unfortunately, participants may still forget stations when the main circuit is in operation. The use of printed circuit training cards to illustrate the exercise to be performed at each station can act as a reminder, however the diagrams need to be large and visible, and the written instructions clear. It is also useful if key coaching points are listed as safety reminders.

The use of assistant teachers and spotters may also assist with effective control, however they will need to be instructed carefully about their role and responsibilities. In reality, assistants are not frequently accessible, so when dealing with inexperienced groups without assistance, it is often easier to reduce the number of stations. Figures 10.3, 10.4 and 10.5 illustrate circuit training formats that are more appropriate for dealing with less experienced groups.

## What circuit formats are available?

There are a number of ways a group can be organised for the main circuit training component. The format selected should be appropriate for the number of stations and the number of participants. If dealing with small groups it is unwise to have a large number of stations with only one person exercising on each. It is advisable to encourage a group of people to perform at each station to assist with group motivation and observation. Five different formats are illustrated in figures 10.1 to 10.5. Some of the advantages and disadvantages for using each of the different formats are also identified.

| Figure 10.1 Square circuit – traditional format | | | |
| --- | --- | --- | --- |
| 1 XXXX | 2 XXXX | 3 XXXX | 4 XXXX |
| XXXX 5 | XXXX 6 | XXXX 7 | XXXX 8 |

**Advantages**
- Can have a large number of exercise stations.
- Can use a variety of equipment.
- Variety of stations will maintain interest and assist motivation.
- Can be very challenging so ideal for fitter participants.
- Ideal for muscular strength and endurance-based circuits.
- Can be used for cardio-vascular and muscular strength and endurance-based sessions, provided exercises are planned effectively, i.e. alternating and spacing stations so that intensity is maintained.

**Disadvantages**
- Harder for the teacher to move around and observe if a large number of stations are used.
- Need assistance to observe when lots of stations.
- Difficult to instruct beginners unless all are placed on the same station, and this may draw the teacher's attention away from the rest of the class.

## Figure 10.2 Lined circuit

| 1 | 2 | 3 | 4 | 5 | 6 | 7 | 8 |
|---|---|---|---|---|---|---|---|
| X | X | X | X | X | X | X | X |
| X | X | X | X | X | X | X | X |
| X | X | X | X | X | X | X | X |
| X | X | X | X | X | X | X | X |
| X | X | X | X | X | X | X | X |
| X | X | X | X | X | X | X | X |
| X | X | X | X | X | X | X | X |

### Advantages

- Works well for cardio-vascular circuits.
- Relatively easy to change stations and maintain work to the music phrase.
- Relatively easy for the teacher to move around and observe.
- Adds variety in a traditional ETM programme.
- Variations can be achieved by planning exercises so that participants have to run to the back after performing a certain number of repetitions of the planned exercise. When the first person is back to the front the whole line can move to the next station. This is also an effective method of timing the circuit.

### Disadvantages

- Difficult, if not impossible, to organise and use equipment for this approach.
- Works less effectively for muscular strength and endurance training, but not impossible or inappropriate.

## Figure 10.3 Corners circuit

```
1                                    2
XXXX                                 XXXX
XXXX                                 XXXX
XXXX                                 XXXX




XXXX                                 XXXX
XXXX                                 XXXX
XXXX                                 XXXX
3                                    4
```

### Advantages

- Works well for cardio-vascular circuits.
- Works well within the cardio-vascular component of a traditional ETM programme.
- Easier to manage due to fewer stations.
- Ideal for small groups.
- Ideal for beginners; fewer exercises to remember and repetition could improve performance.
- Very small groups can perform at one station and the teacher can move around with them to assist performance.

### Disadvantages

- May become too repetitious or boring if the same stations are repeated for a number of circuits.

```
Figure 10.4 Half-split circuit

        1                    2

X X X X X X X X X    X X X X X X X X X X
X X X X X X X X X    X X X X X X X X X X
X X X X X X X X X    X X X X X X X X X X
X X X X X X X X X    X X X X X X X X X X
X X X X X X X X X    X X X X X X X X X X
X X X X X X X X X    X X X X X X X X X X
X X X X X X X X X    X X X X X X X X X X
X X X X X X X X X    X X X X X X X X X X
```

```
Figure 10.5 Command-led circuit

        X        X        X        X
   X        X        X        X        X
        X        X        X        X
   X        X        X        X        X
        X        X        X        X
   X        X        X        X        X
        X        X        X        X
```

### Advantages

- Works well for cardio-vascular circuits.
- Can easily be included as a variation of cardio-vascular training within a traditional ETM session.
- Can work well with one half performing cardio-vascular exercises and the other half performing muscular strength and endurance exercises.
- Easy to manage: only two exercises being performed at the same time.
- Easy to lead and instruct: fewer exercises to explain.
- Ideal for beginners.

### Disadvantages

- May need a spotter to observe one half of the group if complex exercises are used.
- Need to vary the exercises to create interest, prevent boredom and ensure a balanced workout is achieved.

### Advantages

- All participants perform the same activity at the same time.
- Can vary exercises and maintain desired training effect.
- Commands for one exercise only need to be given at any one time.
- No circuit cards are needed: participants follow teacher's commands.
- Effective way of introducing circuit stations as part of a re-warmer.
- Easy to include within a traditional ETM session: participants can be instructed to perform a muscular strength and endurance exercise between cardio-vascular exercises.
- Easy to control large groups.
- Easy to adapt exercises and offer alternatives for different abilities in the same group.

### Disadvantages

- Can be regimental.
- Can be quite strenuous and may be inappropriate for less fit participants: this will depend on which exercises are planned, how they are instructed and whether alternatives are offered.

# How can work time at each station be controlled?

The time spent working on a specific station or exercise can be dictated by either timing each exercise, or specifying the number of repetitions to be performed. Both will require an appropriate work time at each station, and appropriate rest time between stations to be established. The work : rest ratio will need to be appropriate for the target group. Guidelines for appropriate work : rest ratios are provided in table 10.2.

## The time-controlled circuit

There are two approaches to timing a circuit. The first approach is to time the work time and rest time using a stop watch. A disadvantage of this approach is that more attention may be paid to watching the clock rather than participants. However, it does allow for the same time to be spent on each station, and after some experience is gained, it is often possible to estimate the time, rather than 'clock watch'.

Alternatively, the timing can be controlled by a specific station. For example, if Shuttle Runs are used as a station, a set number of runs can be performed before moving on to the next station. A disadvantage of using this approach is that different participants may perform the activity at a different speeds. If some take longer, then the overall work time on each station will vary slightly.

## The repetition-controlled circuit

There are two approaches to controlling the number of repetitions performed. Either the teacher can dictate a set number of repetitions (e.g. 20 repetitions of each exercise), or he/she can allow participants to choose a number (e.g. choose to perform either 8, 12, 16 or 20 repetitions of each exercise).

If the teacher dictates a number of repetitions, the number they suggest may not be appropriate for different abilities. To accommodate this, a range of intensities can be offered, and participants can be advised to select the intensity level at which they can perform the prescribed number of repetitions. However, people may perform at different speeds and some may finish the exercise before others. The same problem can arise if participants are allowed to choose a number of repetitions. The participants will therefore be inactive while they wait for others to finish, and queues may develop at specific stations. The best way to avoid this is to have a control exercise in the middle of the room that participants perform while they wait for the rest of the group to complete their exercise. When the whole group is in the middle of the room, everyone can move on to their next station.

# How can a circuit training session be adapted for different fitness levels?

The intensity of the individual stations can be adapted to suit different requirements by varying the:

- speed of the exercise
- range of motion
- repetitions
- resistance (using longer levers, adding weight etc.).

*Note:* detailed progressions are provided for all the exercises illustrated in chapters 7, 8 and 9.

The intensity of the whole circuit training session can be adapted to accommodate different needs by altering the:

• number of stations
• intensity of the exercises at each station
• time working at each station
• rest time between each station
• number of times the circuit is performed
• rest time between each circuit.

More specific guidelines for adapting the intensity and duration of the circuit to accommodate different fitness levels are outlined in table 10.2.

*Note:* It is recommended that etm teachers who wish to include circuit training within their sessions hold a recognised circuit training qualification. This is to ensure they have a comprehensive knowledge of the different approaches to circuit training that can be adopted.

| Table 10.2 | Adapting the intensity and duration of the circuit for different target groups | | |
|---|---|---|---|
| | *Less fit and specialist groups* | *Intermediate fitness level and general groups* | *Advanced fitness level and sport-specific groups* |
| Overall duration circuit (including warm-up and cool-down) | 45 minutes | 45–60 minutes | 60 minutes |
| Overall intensity of circuit stations | Low | Moderate–High | High |
| Work time on stations *Note:* if muscular strength is a goal then the time will need to be shorter and the intensity higher. | Short | Moderate | Long |
| Rest time between stations *Note:* cardio-vascular circuits will need an active rest. Performing a lower intensity activity between stations should be sufficient. | Long – perform low-intensity activity to allow sufficient recovery | Moderate – perform a moderately intense activity to allow recovery from high-intensity activities | Short rest time needed between more intense activities. Rest periods can be more active: aim for continuous move-ment around circuit |

| Table 10.2 | Adapting the intensity and duration of the circuit for different target groups cont. | | |
|---|---|---|---|
| | Less fit and specialist groups | Intermediate fitness level and general groups | Advanced fitness level and sport-specific groups |
| Approach Note: this may vary to accommodate the fitness goals of the individual/group being trained. | Timed or rep Command-led format is easier to manage | Timed or rep | Timed or rep to tailor programme to meet specific needs |
| Number of stations Note: this may vary depending on the number of participants. | Low (4–8) | Moderate (8–12) | High (10–20) Possibly more, depending on aims of circuit, number of participants and space |
| Number of circuits Note: this will vary depending on the number of stations used. | Low (1–2) | Moderate (1–3) | High (1–4) |
| Appropriate exercises: Note: all the exercises illustrated at the end of chapters 7, 8 and 9. | Compound (working a number of muscles to reduce the number of exercises) | Compound and isolation exercises using equipment | Compound and isolation exercises using equipment |

## Aerobic lined circuit

1. Mambo chasse
2. Power squat
3. Double Grapevine
4. Side lunge
5. Spotty dogs
6. Gazelle leaps
7. Jumping jacks
8. Side squats
9. Back lunge
10. Pony

**Work time:** 50 seconds each station.
**Active rest:** Jog/march to next station 10 seconds
**Total time:** 10 minutes for one circuit. 20 minutes for two circuits.

# DESIGNING A STRETCH AND RELAX PROGRAMME

## 11

## How should a stretch and relax session be structured?

The structure of a specific stretch and relax session should follow the traditional session format: a thorough warm-up and stretch should precede the main workout, and a comprehensive cool-down should conclude the session. An appropriate session structure and suggested content is outlined in table 11.1.

## What activities are appropriate for a stretch and relax session?

All of the stretching exercises illustrated in chapters 5 and 6 are appropriate. These exercises can be performed and repeated throughout the whole session. In addition, the relaxation techniques explained in chapter 6 are effective for releasing muscular tension and can assist with relaxation of the mind.

It should be noted that stretching and relaxation exercises are generally less energetic. It may therefore be necessary to include some controlled range of motion stretches and mobility and pulse raising exercises to keep warm throughout the session. Some exercises that may be appropriate are illustrated and explained in chapter 5. Teachers should select the exercises that flow most naturally and easily into stretch positions. Jerky movements and exercises that do not flow smoothly from one to the other will draw attention away from the desired session aim. That is, they will not promote a relaxed and flowing feel to the movements.

It is also appropriate to include a range of standing and floor based muscular strength and endurances exercises in this type of session. However, too much emphasis on this type of activity will again distract from relaxation. Some of the exercises illustrated in chapter 9 will be appropriate. Once again, to maintain the theme of the session, only those exercises which flow naturally should be used. It is recommended that these exercises be performed at a slower pace with greater emphasis on control and mind and body awareness. The slower pace should help to promote better alignment and will also make the exercises harder (overload).

## What recent developments are there to stretch and relaxation programmes?

Most modern day stretch and relaxation classes incorporate a combination of old and new training techniques from both western and eastern traditions. They blend movements, exercises and postures from Pilates, yoga and tai chi with traditional flexibility, range of motion mobility, core stability training, with isotonic and static muscular strength exercises. Meditation and relaxation techniques are also used in some classes to promote further relaxation, self-awareness and assist with stress management.

A range of exercises/postures used in yoga and pilates are illustrated at the end of this chapter. However, it needs to be recognised that yoga is based on a much deeper spiritual philosophy that cannot be explained in this

| Table 11.1 | Session structure | |
|---|---|
| *Component:* | *Suggested activities:* |
| Posture: | Establish correct posture |
| Breathing: | Raise awareness of the breathe.<br>Can use floating arms and weight transfer. |
| Warm up: | Gentle mobility, pulseraising with range of motion and static stretching. |
| Main workout (standing) | Standing MSE work<br>Standing yoga postures (adapted)<br>Standing tai chi movements (adapted)<br>Standing flexibility work |
| Main workout (floor based) | Floor based MSE work<br>Floor based yoga postures<br>Floor based pilates exercises<br>Core stability exercises<br>Floor based flexibility exercises |
| Cool down | Developmental stretches<br>Relaxation and meditation techniques |

book. Teachers who are interested in this philosophy are recommended to read 'The spiritual teachings of yoga' which is listed as a reference at the back of this book. With this in mind, the exercises illustrated are therefore being suggested as a methods for gaining flexibility, balance and strength. Exercise technique, posture and breathing are all explained. However, the best way to learn effective technique is to work under the supervision of a qualified yoga teacher/practitioner.

Teachers who wish to train further in either yoga or pilates are guided to the training organisations listed at the back of this book.

The emphasis of the session can be adapted by spending more time on specific elements. For example:
- For a greater emphasis on flexibility more developmental stretches can be used.
- For a greater emphasis on relaxation, this component can be lengthened.
- For a greater emphasis on balance, more standing postures and stretches can be used.
- For a greater emphasis on strength, more standing postures, strengthening exercises and core work can be included.

## Posture checks:

- Stand feet hip width apart
- Feet parallel
- Distribute weight between heel bone, big toe & little toe (3 point weight distribution)
- Spread toes
- Align second toe with knee and hip
- Find neutral pelvic position
- Lengthen torso and neck
- Look forwards
- Shoulders relaxed and down
- Shoulder blades squeeze down
- Hands placed by the side, palms facing forward

## Breathing awareness:

Start by focusing awareness on the depth, speed and feeling of the breath. Maintain an open posture.

- Take the breath slightly deeper into the lower rib cage (most people take very shallow breathes into the upper chest area only).
- Keep the breath soft, smooth and rhythmical.
- Find a natural breathing pace.
- Find a natural breathing power (not forcing or straining)
- Let the breath become effortless and allow it to flow freely.
- Allow the breathe to quieten and calm the mind.

# CORE ABDOMINAL EXERCISES

| Ex 1 | Pelvic tilt |
|------|-------------|

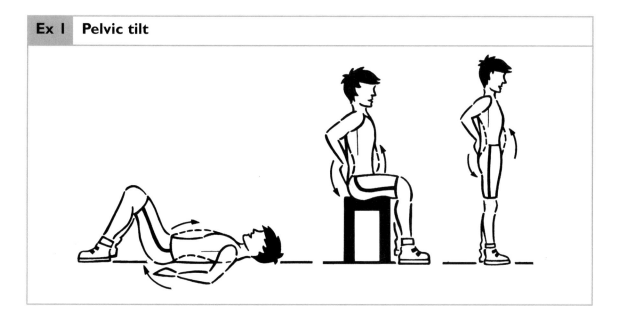

## Purpose

To find the neutral pelvic position. This movement needs to be maintained during abdominal work and other exercises to ensure the lumbar spine does not move excessively.

## Starting position and instructions

**Lying:**
Lie on your back with knees bent, and feet hip width apart. Relax the shoulders and neck. Lengthen the spine.

**Seated:**
Sit on the sitting bones (you can feel these in the middle of each buttock cheek). Sit upright and tall.

**Standing:**
Place your feet hip width apart. Lengthen the spine and stand upright.

## Teaching points

- Tighten the abdominals and buttocks to tilt the pelvis backwards (the pubic bone will press up and the lower back will press to the floor or lower spine flattens).
- Tighten the hips and back to tilt the pelvis forward (the pubic bone lowers and the small of the back hollows).
- Repeat this a few times.
- Find a mid way point between these two movements and hold the pelvis still. This is the neutral pelvic position.
- Control the movement.
- Breathe comfortably throughout.

## Progressions/adaptations/variations

As a variation, perform this exercise seated or standing (keep the spine upright and make sure the movement is isolated and the rest of the body remains still).

## Ex 2  Abdominal hollowing

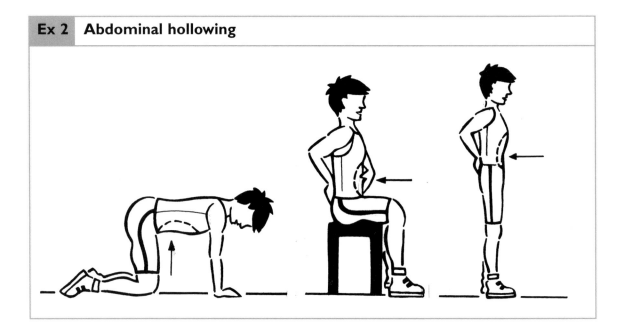

### Purpose

To work the muscles that help to control movement and stabilise the spine.

### Starting position

**Kneeling:**
Place your hands and knees on the floor, shoulder width apart. Find a neutral pelvic position. Tighten the tummy muscles and pull the tummy button towards the spine.

**Seated:**
Sit upright, and lengthen the spine with your feet hip width apart. Find neutral pelvic position.
*NB*: a block can be used to assist with upright and sitting.

**Standing:**
With your feet hip width apart, distribute weight evenly between the heel, big toe and little toe. Find neutral pelvic position.

### Teaching points

- Breathe normally throughout or breathe out when pulling the tummy in.
- Keep the pelvis, spine and shoulders still.
- Make sure the back doesn't flatten.
- Keep the shoulders relaxed and the neck lengthened.
- Elbows unlocked.

### Progressions/adaptations/variations

- The movement of the tummy will be small at first, as the muscles get stronger progress by pulling the tummy in further.
- Perform in a seated position, on a chair and progress to a stability ball.
- Perform standing.

**Rest:** Child pose (if kneeling). *See* page 188.

| Ex 3 | Heel slide |
|---|---|

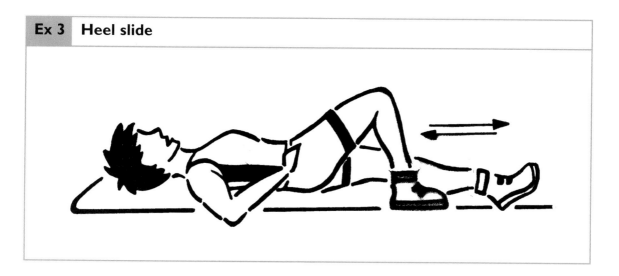

## Purpose

To strengthen the muscles that hold the pelvis still.

## Starting position and instructions

Lie on your back, feet hip width apart. Position the pelvis in a neutral position. Place the hands on the pelvic bones (to monitor movement of the pelvis). The legs need to be able to slide along the floor so perform the exercise without shoes so the socks can slide along the floor. Shoulders need to be relaxed and spine lengthened.

## Teaching points

- Pull the tummy in tight without moving the pelvis (abdominal hollowing).
- Breathe normally throughout the exercise.
- Slide the leg along the floor until you feel the pelvis begin to tilt. At this point pause and slide the leg back to its original position.
- Repeat on the other leg.
- Make sure the legs do not lift off the floor.
- Alternative breathing, on the outward breathe pull the tummy tight and commence leg sliding action. Breathe in, and breathe out, contracting the abdominals to slide the leg back to start position.

## Ex 4  Bridge

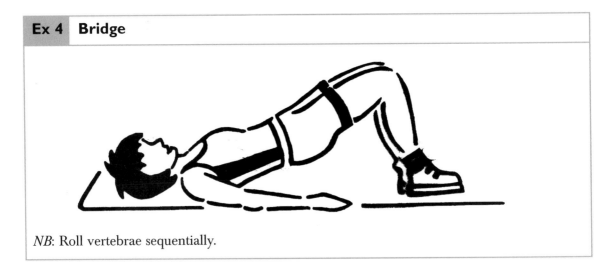

*NB*: Roll vertebrae sequentially.

## Purpose

To further strengthen the muscles that keep the pelvis firm and stable; to mobilise the spine.

## Starting position and instructions

Lie on your back with your knees bent and feet shoulder width apart. Find the neutral pelvic position and maintain this throughout. Relax the shoulders, arms by side and lengthen the spine.

## Teaching points

- Pull the tummy in without moving the pelvis.
- Squeeze the buttock muscles tight and raise the hips from the floor about 4 inches.
- Make sure the back doesn't hollow and the body weight doesn't rise up to the neck.
- Keep the thighs and tummy in line.
- Breathe normally throughout the movement
- Hold for 10 seconds at the top of the movement, breathing normally.
- Control the upward and downward phases of the movement.
- Keep the abdominals in tight throughout.
- Allow the buttock squeeze to initiate and maintain control of the movement.

## Progression

Add a heel raise at the top of the movement. Straighten the knee on one leg taking the weight onto the other leg (keep the pelvis firm).

## Ex 5  Reciprocal reach

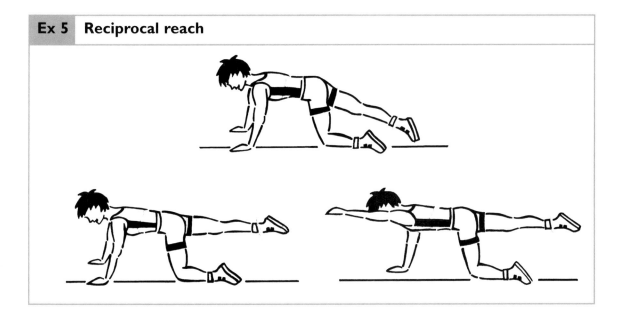

### Level 1 – Leg only to rear
### Level 2 – Leg only to hip height
### Level 3 – Leg and arm to hip height

### Purpose

To strengthen the muscles that maintain the neutral pelvic position and stabilize the spine. To develop balance and control.

### Starting position and instructions

Place your hands and knees on the floor directly underneath the hip and shoulders. Find neutral pelvis. Breathe in and lengthen the spine.

### Level 1.
Breathe out, hollow and tighten the abdominals, sliding the right leg backwards. Breathe in and return the leg to centre. Repeat with other leg.

### Level 2.
Breathe out, hollow and tighten abdominals, slide the right leg backwards and raise to hip height. Breathe in and return the leg to centre.

Repeat with other leg.

### Level 3.
Breathe out, hollow and tighten the abdominals, slide and raise the right leg to hip height and at the same time extend the left arm forwards to shoulder height. Breathe in and return the leg and arm to centre.

### Teaching points

- Maintain neutral pelvis throughout.
- Keep the abdominals tight throughout.
- Keep the spine lengthened.
- Keep the weight evenly distributed through both hands or knees.
- Make sure the back does not dip
- Make sure the pelvis doesn't tilt to one side

Level 3
- Keep the shoulder blade square and the neck and spine lengthened.

**Rest:** Child Pose. (*see* page 188).

# YOGA POSTURES

**Ex 6** | **Mountain pose**

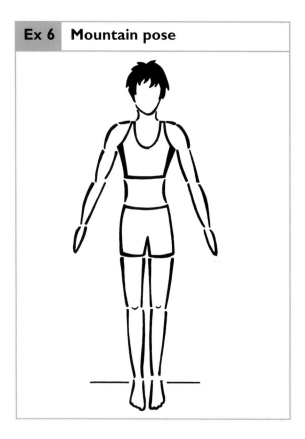

## Purpose

A starting position for all other standing postures. Can be used as a rest, to centre the body between postures.

## Starting position and instructions

- Stand with the feet together or parallel.
- Spine lengthened and shoulders relaxed.
- Neutral pelvic position with abdominals hollowed.

- Weight distributed evenly between the big toes, little toes and heel bones.
- Look straight ahead, with neck lengthened.
- Arms slightly away from the side of the body, lengthening through the fingers.
- Breath naturally.

## Ex 7 | Arm raise and prayer pose

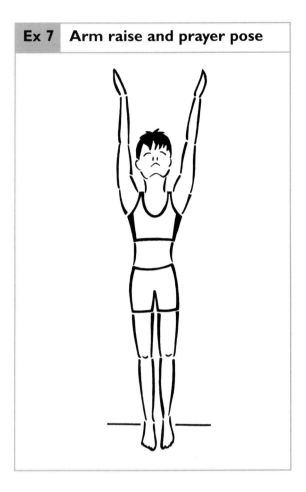

## Purpose

To raise awareness of breathing whilst synchronising movement of the upper body.

## Starting position and instructions

Stand in mountain pose.
- Breathe in, raise the arms out to the side of the body and reaching above the head, look up slightly.
- Breathe out, placing the palms together in a prayer position and lower the arms to level with the chest, look straight ahead.
- Breathe in, raise the arms up into a prayer position above the head, look up slightly.

- Breathe out and lower the arms back down to the sides of the body, look straight ahead.
- Rest and repeat.

## Teaching points

- Maintain neutral pelvis
- Keep the spine lengthened.
- Keep the shoulders relaxed and neck long.

**Rest:** Mountain pose (*see* page 176).

## Ex 8 | Chair pose

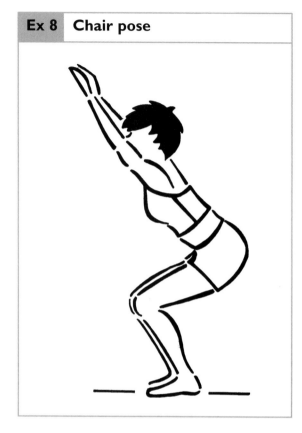

### Purpose

A strong, dynamic movement that will raise the heart rate, increase circulation and warm the body when performed repeatedly and rhythmically. Will also strengthen the muscles of the thighs and buttocks (Quadriceps, Hamstrings and Gluteals)

### Starting position and instructions

- Start in Mountain pose, feet parallel at hip width. Spread the weight evenly between the feet.
- Breathe in, lengthen the body
- Breathe out and simultaneously bend the knees to 90 degrees and raise the arms in front of the body until they are close to the ears. Hands should touch lightly in prayer position.
- Hold for as long as comfortable, breathing naturally.
- Lift out of the position on an outward breath (exhalation)
- Rest and repeat.

### Teaching points

- Keep the abdomen hollow,
- Look forward, and slightly up when arms raise.
- Maintain the length of the spine.
- Keep the neck long and shoulders relaxed.
- Make sure you don't hold your breath.
- Keep both feet firmly on the floor, weight spread evenly.

### Adaptation

- Bend to a lesser angle that can be achieved comfortably.
- Raise the arms to a lower height.

**Rest:** Mountain pose (*see* page 176).

## Ex 9 — Gazing pose (and Intense stretch pose)

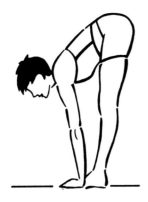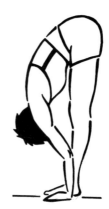

### Purpose

Lengthens the spine and the muscles at the back of the thigh and hip (Hamstrings and Gluteals).

### Starting Position and Instructions

- Start in mountain pose, feet parallel at hip width. Spread the weight evenly between the feet.
- Breathe in, lengthen the body and tighten and hollow the abdomen.
- Breathe out and bend forward at the hip/pelvis and place the hands on the floor at the outside of the feet (or hold the back of the calves).
- Inhale and lift the head to gaze forward, lengthening the spine and relaxing the shoulders. Hold for as long as comfortable, breathing naturally.
- To release, breath in, bend the legs and raise the arms to the side of the ears, palms together moving into chair pose.
- Breathe out, straighten the legs, lower the arms into mountain pose.
- Rest and repeat.

- You can progress into the intense stretch pose here if you wish.
- Exhale and bend the arms, extending the spine into a longer position towards the thighs.
- Keep the neck and shoulders relaxed.
- Breath naturally.

### Teaching points

- Keep the spine lengthened.
- Keep the shoulders relaxed and open the chest.
- Maintain hollow abdominals
- Keep the knees unlocked by maintaining an upward pull of the front thigh muscles.
- Keep the weight spread evenly between the feet.

### Progression and Adaptation

- Bend the knees to move into the forward bend. Keep the knees slightly bent during the forward bend, easing the legs a little straighter to a position that feels comfortable.
- To progress, add intense stretch pose.

**Rest:** Mountain pose (*see* page 176).

## Ex 10 | Crane pose

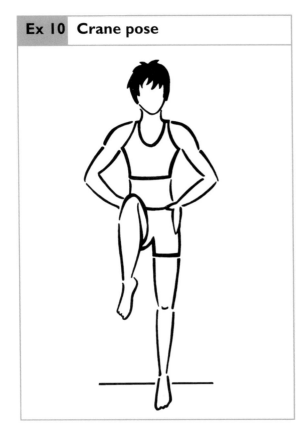

### Purpose

To develop balance and stability. It is a starting point before attempting to perform other more advanced standng postures.

### Starting position and instructions

- Stand with feet parallel and ankles as close together as possible. Arms at the side of the body.
- The body weight should be distributed evenly between the big toe, little toe and heels of both feet.
- The arches of the feet should be lifted to prevent the ankles rolling
- Tighten the thigh muscles, drawing the knee cap upwards.
- Take the body weight onto one leg and place the hands on the pelvic bones.
- Raise the other leg so that the knee is slightly higher than the hip and the foot is in line under the hip.
- Lower the leg and repeat on the other side.

### Teaching points

- Maintain a neutral pelvic position.
- Keep the spine lengthened and the abdominals tight (abdominal hollowing).
- Keep the chest open and the neck lengthened.
- Breathe comfortably throughout.

### Adaptation

Lift the leg to hip height or lower if flexibility is limited.

**Rest:** Mountain Pose.

## Ex 11   Forward stretch

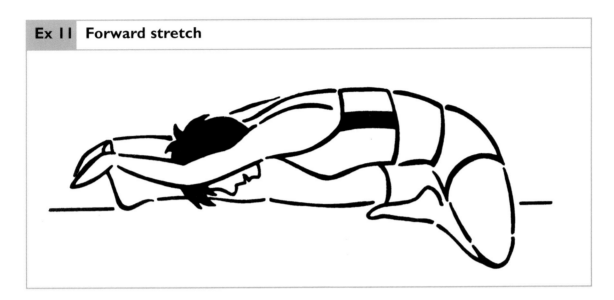

## Purpose

Relaxes and lengthens the spine and lengthens the muscles at the back of the thigh (hamstrings)

## Starting positions and instructions

Sit in the staff pose.
Bend one leg and place the sole of the foot on the inside of the thigh as close to the pubic bone as comfortable.

- Breathe in, opening the chest and lengthening the spine.
- Breathe out and bend forward at the hip, reaching the hands forward to take hold of the foot.
- Breathe in, lengthening the spine and neck, lifting the chin slightly.
- Breathe out, bend the arms and lengthen forward further into the stretch.
- Breathe in, lengthening the spine and easing the crown of the head forwards.

- Hold the position for as long as comfortable, breathing naturally.
- Breath in, to lengthen out of the stretch and back into staff pose.
- Rest and repeat on the other leg.

## Teaching points

- Keep the spine lengthened and the shoulders relaxed.
- Lengthen and hollow the abdomen.
- Chest should remain wide and relaxed.

## Adaptation

Place the leg out to the side of the body at 90 degrees
Reach towards the toes, but place the hands in a position that is comfortable.

**Rest:** Staff pose (*see* page 183).

## Ex 12  Tree pose

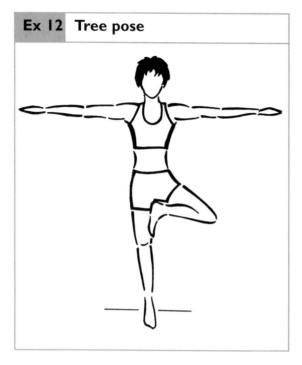

### Purpose

To develop balance and stability and opens up the hip joint. Helps to focus the mind.

### Starting position and instructions

- Stand with feet parallel and ankles as close together as possible.
- The body weight should be distributed evenly between the big toe, little toe and heels of both feet.
- The arches of the feet should be lifted to prevent the ankles rolling.
- Tighten the thigh muscles, drawing the knee cap upwards.
- Take the body weight onto one leg.
- Raise the other leg and take hold of the ankle.
- Place the foot on the raised leg on the inside thigh of the supporting leg.

- Take the arms to the side of the body, level with the shoulders and parallel to the floor.
- Turn the knee outwards on the bent leg to open up the hip.
- Lower the leg and repeat on the other side.

### Teaching points

- Maintain a neutral pelvic position.
- Keep the spine lengthened and the abdominals tight (abdominal hollowing).
- Keep the chest open and the neck lengthened.
- Breathe comfortably throughout.

### Adaptation

Place the leg slightly lower, either above or below the knee to accommodate limited flexibility.

**Rest:** Mountain pose (*see* page 176).

## Ex 13  Staff pose

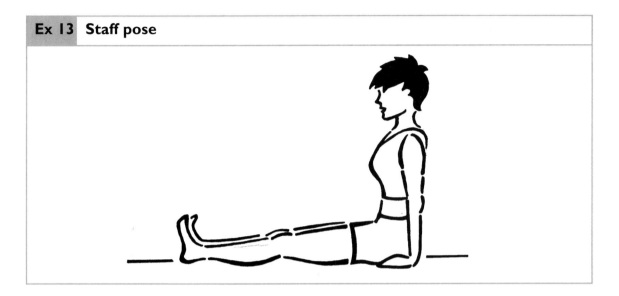

## Purpose

Basic sitting position that prepares for other seated postures. Challenging when performed correctly and held for a few breaths.

## Starting position and instructions

Sit upright, fully onto the sitting bones with the legs out straight. Place the hands on the floor at the side of the hips. Spread the toes pressing the balls of the feet lightly away from the body.

## Teaching points

- Lengthen and hollow the abdominals.
- Maintain a neutral pelvis by keeping the core muscles strong, yet soft.
- Keep the shoulders relaxed and spine lengthened.
- Keep the knees unlocked.

## Adaptation

Sit with the back against a wall to assist with support the spine.

**Rest:** Bend the knees and let the body rest forward over the thighs.

## Ex 14  Easy Boat pose

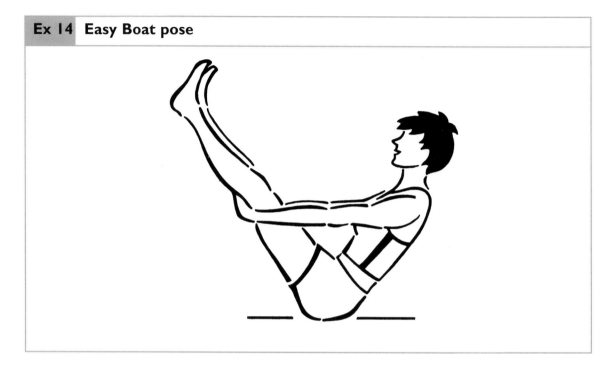

## Purpose

Develops balance. Strengthens the legs and core stabilisers.

## Starting position and instructions

Sit on the floor with legs bent, and the spine lengthened. Breathe in, taking the weight backwards onto your buttocks, with your feet off the floor, and wrap the hands around the back of the thighs. Breathe out and extend the knees. Breathe in and bend the knees again. Breathe out and place the feet on the floor.

## Teaching points

- Maintain a neutral pelvis.
- Keep the spine lengthened, shoulders relaxed and ribcage open.
- Keep the abdominals tightened and hollow.

## Progression and adaptation

- To make the exercise easier, keep the knees bent at 90 degrees.
- To make the exercise harder, lengthen the arms to the side of the legs.

**Rest:** Staff pose or rest for Staff pose (*see* page 183).

## Ex 15 Open pose

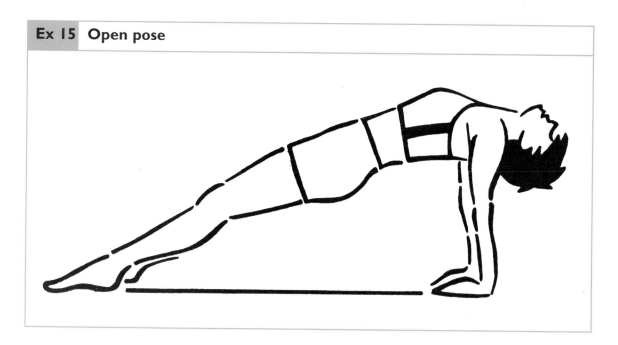

### Purpose

Lengthens the muscles of the chest (pectorals) and the forearm.

### Starting positions and instructions

- Sit upright in Staff pose.
- Breathe in and lean back, sliding the hands backwards on the floor behind you. Keep the fingers facing forward.
- Breathe out and straighten the arms, pressing the palms down.
- Breathe in and lift and open the chest, hollowing the back slightly.
- Hold for as long as comfortable, breathing naturally.
- Breath out to return to Staff pose.
- Rest and repeat.

### Teaching points

Keep the shoulders relaxed and the spine lengthened. Keep the abdominals hollowed.

### Progression and Adaptation

- Bend the knees to adapt the pose.
- To progress the pose, keeping the legs bent, lift the buttocks of the floor and press the hip upward, maintaining neutral pelvis.
- To progress further, with straight legs, raise the buttocks off the floor, so the whole body weight is supported between the hands and feet. Keep your body straight.

**Rest:** Staff pose or rest for Staff pose (*see* page 183).

## Ex 16 | Cat pose

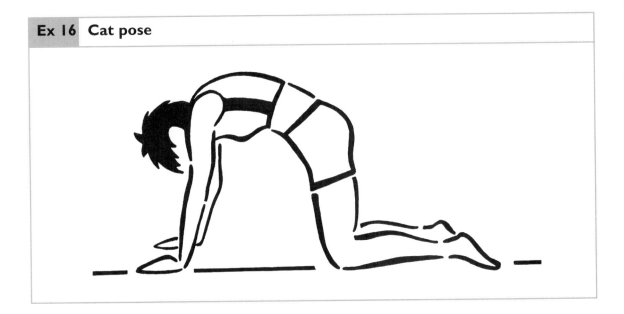

### Purpose

To focus awareness on synchronisation of breathing whilst moving the spine. Will improve mobility of the spine.

### Starting position and instructions

Position yourself on your hands and knees, with your hands underneath the shoulders, and your knees underneath the hips. Breathe in, hollow the spine slightly, tilting the tailbone in the air. Breathe out, tighten the abdominals and tuck the tailbone underneath, rounding the spine. Repeat.

### Teaching points

- Keep the neck and shoulders relaxed and lengthened.
- Keep the weight spread evenly between the hands and knees.
- Keep the movement slow and controlled.
- Be aware of moving only to a comfortable range of motion within the limitations of your own body.

**Rest:** Child pose (*see* page 188).

## Ex 17 Dog pose

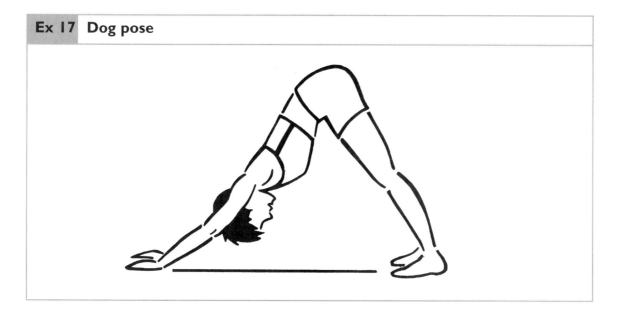

## Purpose

To focus awareness on breathing. Lengthens the muscles at the back of the legs, buttocks and lower back. Strengthens the upper body.

## Starting position and instructions

- Position yourself on your hands and knees.
- Keep the hands underneath the shoulders, weight distributed evenly between fingers, thumbs and balls of the hands.
- Keep the knees underneath the hips.
- Place the toes and balls of the feet on the floor.
- Breathe in, hollow the spine slightly, tilting the tailbone in the air (Cat pose).
- Breathe out, tighten the abdominals and straighten the legs with the sitting bones pointing towards the ceiling (Dog pose).
- Repeat.

## Teaching points

- Keep the neck, shoulders and head relaxed and lengthened.
- Keep the weight spread evenly between the hands and knees/hands and feet.
- Keep the movement slow and controlled.
- Be aware of moving only to a comfortable range of motion within the limitations of your own body.
- Keep the spine relaxed and lengthened.

## Adaptation

Keep the knees slightly bent during the Dog pose to reduce the stretch on the muscles at the back of the leg.

**Rest:** Child pose (*see* page 188).

## Ex 18 Child pose

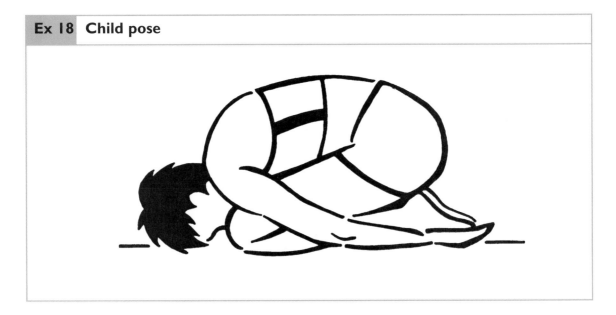

### Purpose

Provides a restful position for the whole body. Can be used as a rest/relaxation between cat and dog pose or any other postures and exercises where the upper and lower body are used simultaneously and are bearing the body weight.

### Starting position and instructions

- Start on the hands and knees.
- Slide the buttocks back to rest on the heels with the chest resting on the thighs.
- Slide the hands down to the side of the body.
- Hold for as long as comfortable.

### Teaching points

- Breathe comfortably throughout.
- Relax the shoulders and neck.
- Keep the spine lengthened.
- Tighten and hollow the abdomen.

### Adaptation

- Form two fists with the hands and place one on top of the other and underneath the forehead to support the head and neck.
- Alternatively, lengthen the arms in front of the body.
- Keep the buttocks slightly away from the buttocks if flexibility of the spine is limited.

# RELAXATION AND MEDITATION POSTURES

## 20 Sitting pose

### Purpose

Opens the hips, strengthens the back and core muscles. Prepares for meditation and awareness of the mind.

### Starting position and instructions

- Sit with the legs crossed one in front of the other, in line with the pubic bone.
- Sit fully onto the sitting bones.
- Lengthen the spine and relax the shoulders.
- Position the hands either:
  a) On the lap with one palm up resting on top of the other palm, arms relaxed.
  b) One hand resting on each knee.

### Teaching points

- Maintain a neutral pelvic position.
- Breathe naturally.
- Alternate the leg that is in front (each time you sit in this position) to ensure equal opening of the hips.

### Adaptation

- Sit against a wall to support the spine.
- Sit in a chair with the feet firmly on the floor and the spine lengthened.

## 21 Lying (Corpse) pose

### Purpose

Promotes relaxation of the body and focuses the attention of the mind on the body in preparation for meditation.

### Starting position and instructions

- Lie on your back with legs straight, arms at the side of the body and palms facing upwards.
- Lengthen the neck and draw the shoulders away from the ears.
- Relax the hips and lower back.
- Relax the legs and allow the feet to roll outwards.

### Teaching points

- Notice how the body contacts the floor.
- Become aware of the body, where tension is stored, where there is tightness – allow the body to let go and to relax.
- Allow the breath to become deeper and softer, effortless.
- Allow the mind to feel peaceful.

### Alternative

Lie in any position that feels comfortable. However, corpse position allows the body to be most open.

## Ex 22  Lying arm raise

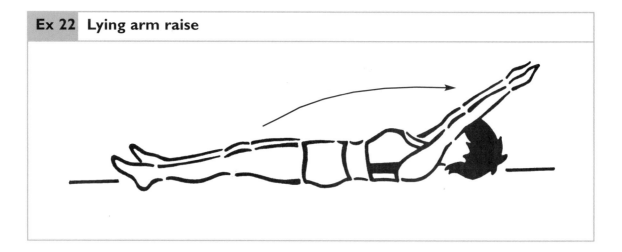

### Purpose

To focus awareness on the synchronisation of breathing with movement of the arms, chest and abdomen.

### Starting position and instructions

- Lie on your back (corpse pose).
- Breathe in, whilst raising the arms over the head till they reach the floor.
- Breathe out, whilst returning the arms to the starting position.

### Teaching points

- Maintain a neutral pelvis.
- Hollow the abdomen.
- Keep the body lengthened and relaxed.
- Keep the rib cage open.
- Make the movements slow and controlled.
- Focus awareness on the breath and the control of the movement.

## Ex 23  Lying leg raise

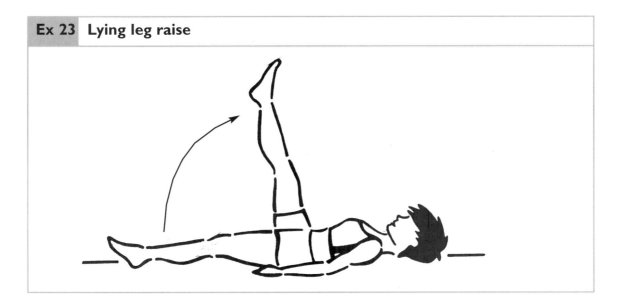

### Purpose

To focus awareness on synchronisation of the breathing with movement of the lower limbs.

### Starting position and instructions

- Lie on your back (corpse pose).
- Find neutral pelvic position.
- Breathe in, keeping the spine long and chest open.
- Breathe out, hollow and tighten the abdomen and raise one leg to a comfortable height.
- Breathe in, lower the leg to the floor.
- Repeat, lifting the other leg as you breathe out and lowering the leg as you breathe in.

### Teaching points

- Maintain a neutral pelvis throughout.
- Hollow and tighten the abdomen.
- Keep the body lengthened and relaxed.
- Keep the rib cage open.
- Make the movements slow and controlled.
- Focus awareness on the breath and the control of the movement.

### Adaptation

Perform the exercise with a bent knee, rather than a straight leg. This will reduce the weight and length of the leverage movement.

## Relaxation script for mind and body class

- Sit or lie in a comfortable position. (*See* relaxation and meditation postures).
- Allow your body to relax and lengthen.
- Allow the muscles to soften.
- Focus your awareness on your breathing.
- Notice the depth and pace of your breathing.
- Allow your breath to become slower, softer and deeper.
- Take your minds awareness to your body, starting with the feet.
- Allow the feet to soften and relax, let go of any tension.
- Allow the ankle joint to open and relax.
- Feel the calf muscles and muscles at the front of the shin soften.
- Take a deeper breathe and on the outward breathe allow the lower leg to relax and soften even further.
- Take your minds awareness to the knee joint.
- Allow the knee joint to open and relax.
- Feel the muscles at the front of the thigh soften.
- Feel the muscles at the back of the thigh lengthen and relax.
- Take a deeper breathe and on the outward breathe allow the whole of the legs to relax and let go.
- Focus your minds awareness to the hip joint.
- Allow the hip joint to open up and relax.
- Feel the buttock muscles relax and soften.
- Feel the muscles around the hip release and open.
- Focus your minds awareness on the spine.
- Start at the base of the spine and be mindful of each vertebrae up to the skull.
- Feel each vertebrae open up.
- Allow the muscles around the vertebrae (spine) to relax and lengthen.
- Allow all the tension to ease away.
- Allow the shoulder blades to separate and open up.
- Take a deep breath and allow the whole spine to lengthen and relax.
- Focus on the abdominal muscles.
- Allow them to release.
- Notice how the breath fills the abdominal area.
- Observe the abdomen rising and falling with each breath.
- Notice the rib cage and the breast bone.
- Feel the muscles around the ribs relax.
- Allow the breath to become slower and deeper.
- Allow the ribs and the breastbone to soften.
- Focus your awareness on the shoulder joint.
- Allow the shoulder joint to open up and relax.
- Feel the muscles of the upper arm lengthen and relax.
- Notice the elbow joint.
- Feel the elbow joint relaxing and opening.
- Feel the muscles of the forearm relax and soften.
- Notice the wrists and the hands.
- Allow the tension to ease away.
- Allow the fingers to curl open and the tension to float away.
- Focus your minds awareness on the head.
- Allow each of the facial muscles to soften and relax.
- Feel the jaw relax.
- Feel the tongue soften.
- Feel the lips gently touching and forming a soft smile.
- Allow the cheek bones to relax.
- Notice the eye sockets relaxing.
- Allow the forehead to relax.
- Any tension just easing away.
- Feel your body soften.
- Allow your body to feel light and relaxed.
- Take your minds awareness back to your breathing.
- Focus on slower, deeper breathing.
- With every breath allow the body to relax further.

- Allow a feeling of peace and calm to spread through your whole body.

*Note*: On completion of relaxation a silent period can be allowed for individual mindfulness/meditation.

To finish relaxation and meditation:
- Bring the minds attention back to the room and notice the sounds you hear around you.
- Gently move the toes and the feet.
- Feel the energy move through the legs.
- Gently move the fingers and hands.
- Feel the energy move through the arms.
- Gently move your head from the right side to the left.

- Feel the energy move through the head.
- Bend the knees, placing the feet on the floor.
- Allow the legs to bend over towards the right, hold for 10 seconds.
- Return legs to centre and allow them to lower to the left, hold for 10 seconds.
- Return the legs to centre.
- Hug the knees to the chest and curl the head towards the knees.
- In your own time, roll onto one side and gradually raise your body to a standing position.
- Shake out the whole body slowly and steadily.

| Table 11.2 | Warm up for mind and body workout | |
|---|---|---|
| **Timing** | **Exercise Description and Purpose** | **Alternative** |
| 1 × 8 R<br>1 × 8 L | Shoulder lifts<br>*Mobilise shoulders* | |
| 1 × 16 | Shoulder rolls<br>*Mobilise shoulders* | |
| 1 × 16 | Spine twists<br>*Spine mobility* | |
| 1 × 16 | Side bends<br>*Spine mobility* | |
| 2 × 16 | Knee lifts<br>*Hip mobility and pulse raise* | With all mobility movements adapt range of motion to suit individual ability. |
| 3–4 minutes approx | *Combination 1:*<br>Mountain pose<br>Arm raise and Prayer pose<br>Adapted chair pose/swing arms by side | Adapt range of motion to suit individual ability. |
| All 10 sec hold | *Tricep stretch*<br>*Pectoral stretch*<br>*Lat stretch* | |
| | *Total time = 8 minutes* | |

| Table 11.3 | Main workout (mind and body): Standing – kneeling – prone lying postures, stretches and MSE work. | |
|---|---|---|
| *Timing* | *Exercise Description and Purpose* | *Alternative* |
| | Mountain pose | |
| 30 secs | Tree pose – right | See adaptations for tree pose |
| | Mountain pose | |
| 30 secs | Tree pose – left | Hold pose longer to increase mindfulness |
| 10 secs | Quad stretch – right | |
| 10 secs | Quad stretch – left | |
| 3-4 minutes | *Develop combination 1:* Mountain pose Arm raise and prayer pose Perform Chair pose Add Gazing pose | Add intense stretch pose after gazing pose for more flexible participants<br><br>Use adaptation to gazing pose for less flexible. Place hands on knees. |
| | Transition to floor | Walk hands forward to floor |
| 30 secs | Dog pose | Hold longer if comfortable. |
| 30 secs | Cat pose | Hold longer if comfortable |
| 2-3 minutes | Cat and dog pose combination | |
| 1 minute | Child pose | Adapt child pose – see exercise instructions |
| 2-2 × 16 reps | Press ups | Box or _ or full press up to suit ability |
| 10-20 seconds | Hover press up (holding in downward movement phase) | |
| 10 seconds | Rectus abdominus stretch | Adaptation from cobra position – not illustrated |
| 30 seconds | Child pose | |
| 10-30 seconds | Plank | Adapt to suit individuals strength. Lying, _ or full. Can vary length of hold. |
| 2-2 × 20 reps | Back extensions | Use single time and decrease reps as needed. |
| 2-2 × 20 reps | Prone flyes | Use single time and decrease reps as needed. |
| 2 minutes | Reciprocal reach | Adapt to single reach of either arm or leg to suit individuals. |
| 1 minute | Child pose | |
| | Total time = 20 minutes | |
| | *Total time = 8 minutes* | |

| Table 11.4 | Main workout (mind and body): Supine lying – postures/stretches/MSE work | |
|---|---|---|
| *Timing* | *Exercise Description and Purpose* | *Alternative* |
| 1 minute | Bridge (move slowly into and out of position) | |
| 3-1 × 8 reps<br>1-3 × 8 reps | Curl up | |
| 1-1 × 16 reps | Oblique curl – x tone | |
| 30 seconds | Staff pose | |
| 30-60 seconds | Forward reach | |
| 20 seconds | Staff pose | |
| 20 seconds | Easy boat | |
| 20 seconds | Staff pose | |
| 30 seconds | Open pose | |
| | *Total time = 10 minutes* | |

| Table 11.5 | Lesson plans: Cooldown (mind and body): Seated to standing – postures/stretches. | |
|---|---|---|
| *Timing* | *Exercise Description and Purpose* | *Alternative* |
| 30 seconds | Wide leg adductor stretch | Adapt to soles of feet together adductor stretch |
| 10 seconds<br>R and L | Tricep stretch | |
| 10 seconds<br>R and L | Oblique stretch | |
| 20 seconds | Seated erector spinae stretch | |
| | *Can include relaxation and meditation here. Select any position.* | *Time can be adapted to suit needs of class.* |
| 20 seconds | Transition to standing | |
| 15 seconds<br>R and L | Gastrocnemius (calf stretch) | |
| 1 minute | Mountain pose<br>Arm raise and prayer pose | |
| | *Total time = 6 minutes without relaxation/meditation* | |

# CORE STABILITY BALL TRAINING

## 12

There is a numerous amount of equipment being manufactured to assist teachers and personal trainers develop participants functional and core stability. One of the most popular pieces of equipment is the stability ball (swiss ball).

There are many benefits for using a core stability ball, provided the exercises are performed safely and the individual has a good base level of sore stability. These benefits include:

| Table 12.1 | The core muscles | |
|---|---|---|
| Muscle name | Position | Function |
| Rectus abdominus | Front abdomen<br>Runs from lower ribs to pubic bone | Flex the spine |
| Internal and external obliques | Side of trunk.<br>Run diagonally from pelvis to ribs | Internal – stabilise the spine<br>External – rotate and laterally flex the spine |
| Transverses abdominus | Runs horizontally around the abdomen from the pelvis and the spinal extensors to the Rectus Abdominus. | Supports the spine and pulls in the abdominals |
| Quadratus lumborum | Side and back of the trunk.<br>Runs from the ribcage to the pelvis. | Stabilises the spine when an external force tries to bend the spine sideways (eg. Carrying a suitcase) |
| Pelvic floor | Positioned like a hammock underneath the pelvis.<br>Runs from pubic bone to coccyx. | Works in partnership with other abdominal muscles. |
| Multifidus | A deeper muscle.<br>Attaching to the transverses muscle and the spinous processes. | Extends individual sections of the spine. |
| Erector spinae | Runs down the back of the spine.<br>Attaching from the base of the skull to the sacrum (base of the spine), pelvis and thorax. | Extends the spine and rotates the thoracic Spine. |

- Improved strength of core muscles.
- Improved balance.
- Improved appearance of abdominals (flatter abdominal area).
- Reduced back pain.
- Improved postural alignment.
- Improved functional movement patterns.

This chapter identifies the core muscles and their function (*see* table 12.1). It also illustrates and explains a range of exercises and provides a basic session structure (*see* table 12.2).

## What are the core muscles?

The core muscles are those that surround the middle section of the body from the ribcage to the pelvis. Collectively, they hold the trunk firm providing a strong and stable base from which other movements of the limbs can be performed safely and effectively. All daily activities (lifting, walking, sitting, carrying, sport and exercise)

require these muscles to be strong.

## How should a stability ball session be structured?

As with all other training sessions, there must be adequate warm up before the main workout and adequate cool down to end the session.

## What safety issues need to be considered?

A primary safety issue before introducing the use of the stability ball is that individuals are able to hold correct technique and alignment on a stable surface. Working on the core stability ball provides an unstable surface. This makes it harder for participants to maintain correct alignment.

| Table 12.2 Session structure | |
|---|---|
| *Component* | *Suggested activities* |
| Standing posture check and abdominal hollowing: | See posture check/stretch section |
| Warm up (free-standing): | Mobility, pulseraising and stretching. |
| Seated posture check and abdominal hollowing. | See instructions – how to sit on the ball. |
| Main workout (seated on ball) | A range of muscular strength and endurance exercises seated on the ball. |
| Main workout (lying on the ball) | Prone/front lying MSE work<br>Supine/back lying MSE work |
| Lying posture check and abdominal hollowing. | See instructions for exercise 11.1 pelvic tilt. |
| Main workout<br>(Lying on floor with feet on ball) | Supine/back lying MSE work |
| Cool down | Developmental and maintenance stretches |

## General safety considerations:

- Make sure the ball is inflated to the correct height for the user (do not over inflate the ball).
- Ensure the ball is placed on a stable surface.
- Ensure there are no sharp objects on the floor around the ball.
- Keep the ball away from direct heat.
- Allow a space of 4 square metres around the ball to exercise safely.
- Check manafacturers guidelines to find out how much weight the ball can withstand. Most balls can hold up to 300kg).

## Ball height

Core stability balls come in different sizes, usually 55cm, 65cm and 75cm. The correct height of ball for an individual is determined by their height and lever length. As a general guideline, an individuals ball height can be found by finding their height in centimetres and subtracting 100. This will be accurate within a 5 centimetre margin.

For example:
168 centimetres (height) – 100 = 68 centimetre (ball height)

## Starting positions and correct posture

### Seated on ball

For all seated exercises:
- Neutral pelvis.
- Abdominal hollowed.
- Feet hip width apart.
- Spine lengthened.
- Breathe out on lifting phase
- Shoulders relaxed and down.
- Look forward.
- Ears, shoulders and hips in line.

## Lying on floor with feet on ball

For all floor lying exercises:
- Maintain neutral pelvis.
- Abdominals hollowed.
- Spine lengthened.
- Shoulders relaxed.
- Breathe out on lifting phase.

## Lying on Ball (back and front)

For all exercises lying on the ball:
- Maintain neutral pelvis.
- Abdominals hollowed.
- Spine lengthened.
- Shoulders relaxed.
- Breathe out on lifting phase.

## Seated on ball

- Hold dumbbells at side of ball.
- Keep elbows close to sides.
- Bend and straighten arms.
- Keep elbows unlocked.

| Ex I | Bicep curl |
|------|------------|

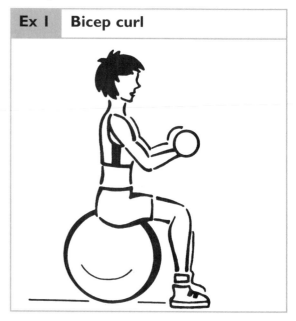

| Ex 2 | **Overhead dumbbell triceps press** |
|---|---|

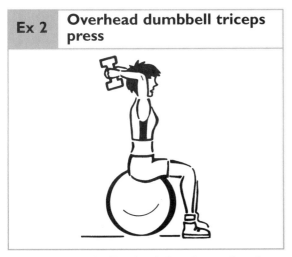

- Hold Dumbbell in both hands overhead.
- Relax shoulders away from ears.
- Bend and straighten elbows, lowering dumbbell behind head.
- Elbows unlocked.
- Elbows stay close to head.

| Ex 4 | **Dumbbell lateral raise** |
|---|---|

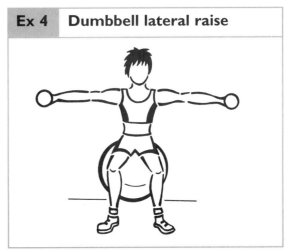

- Hold dumbbells at side of body.
- Raise dumbbells level with shoulders.
- Elbows and wrists in line.
- Elbows unlocked.

| Ex 3 | **Dumbbell shoulder press** |
|---|---|

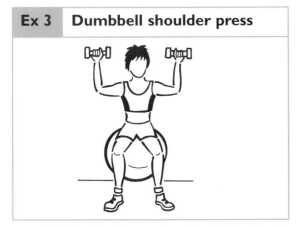

- Hold dumbbells at side of body level with shoulders.
- Relax shoulders.
- Elbows at 90 degree angle
- Extend arms overhead and lower down under control.
- Elbows unlocked.
- Wrist firm and knuckles face upwards.

| Ex 5 | **Dumbbell front raise** |
|---|---|

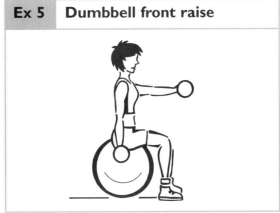

- Hold dumbbells at side of body.
- Alternately raise one hand and then the other in front of the body to shoulder height.
- Keep shoulder blades squeezing lightly back and downwards.
- Elbows unlocked.

| Ex 6 | Leg extension |
|---|---|

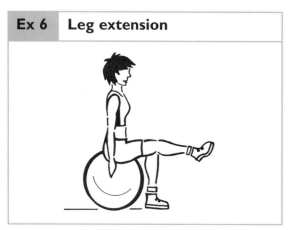

- Feet hip width apart.
- Maintain tight abdominals.
- Raise one leg straight, knee unlocked.
- Keep weight central.

| Ex 8 | Sit up and twist |
|---|---|

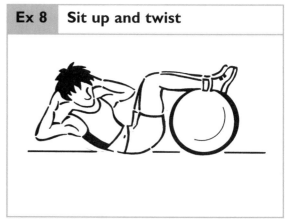

- Hands at side of head.
- Curl head and shoulders off the floor, rotating shoulder towards opposite knee.
- Lower under control

## Lying on floor with feet on ball

| Ex 7 | Sit up |
|---|---|

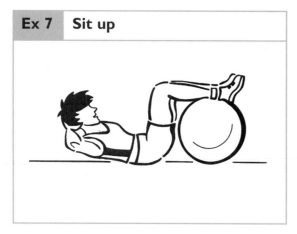

- Hands at side of head.
- Curl head and shoulders off the floor and lower back down under control.

| Ex 9 | Bridge (feet on ball) |
|---|---|

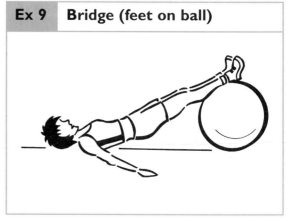

- Feet or calves on ball.
- Squeeze buttocks to raise pelvis off the floor – hold for 5–10 seconds
- Curl down, one vertebrae at a time.
- Breathe naturally throughout.

### Ex 10  Bridge and roll

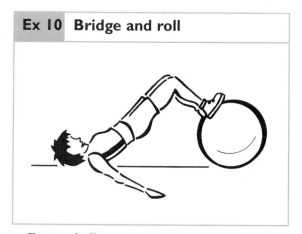

- Feet on ball.
- Bend knees and roll ball towards the buttocks.
- Extend knees and roll ball away from buttocks.
- Keep the buttocks tight throughout.

## Lying on Ball (back)

### Ex 11  Sit up

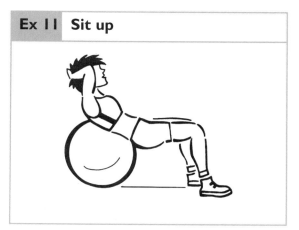

- Lying with back on the ball, feet firmly on floor at hip width.
- Raise and lower the body.
- Take care not to arch the back.

### Ex 12  Sit up twist

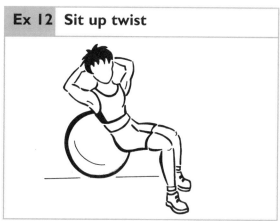

- Lying with back on the ball, feet firmly on floor at hip width.
- Raise and lower the head and shoulders, rotating towards one side.
- Lower under control.
- Repeat raising to other side.

### Ex 13  Dumbbell chest press

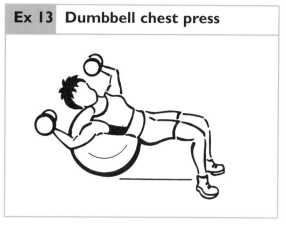

- Lying with your back on ball, feet at hip width and firmly on floor.
- Raise dumbbells above chest, palms inwards.
- Lower dumbbells out to the side of body and level with the mid chest.
- Elbows and wrists in alignment, knuckles face up, palms face towards the feet.
- Raise back up under control, elbows unlocked.

## Ex 14 Lying on ball (front)

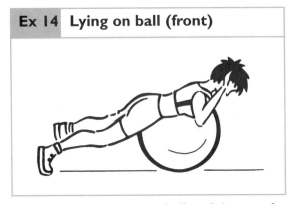

- Lying with tummy on ball and feet on the floor.
- Hands either on buttocks or at side of head.
- Raise the body upwards and lower down under control.

## Ex 16 Prone flyes (prone lying on ball)

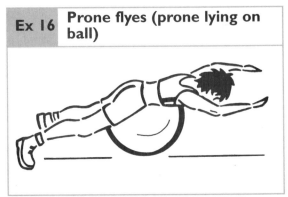

- Lying with tummy on ball and feet on the floor.
- Hands out to the side of the body close to the floor
- Raise arms to level with shoulder girdle.
- Initiate the movement by squeezing the muscles between the shoulder blades.
- Lower under control.

## Ex 15 Press ups

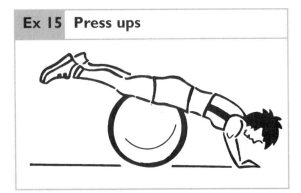

- With either the front thighs or feet on ball.
- Hands on the floor, a shoulder width and a half apart, shoulders in advance of thumbs.
- Lower the chest towards the floor.
- Raise under control, elbows unlocked.

## Ex 17 Gluteal raise

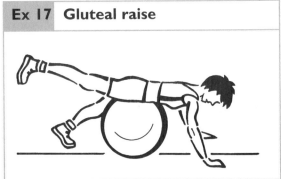

- Lying with the tummy on the ball, hands and feet on the floor.
- Raise and lower one leg to hip height by squeezing the buttock muscles.
- Keep the knee unlocked.
- Control the movement.

*NB*: There are many more advanced exercises that can be performed on the ball. These are not illustrated. It is recommended that teachers attend training to gain further knowledge about working with the ball before attempting more advanced exercises.

| Table 12.3 | General mobility and pulse raising for core ball class – (Mixed ability) | | |
|---|---|---|---|
| Timing | Exercise Description and Purpose | Alternative For less skilled | Progression For more skilled |
| 1 × 16 | Slow plie squats *Knee mobility & pulseraising* | Smaller bend | Deeper bend and increase repetitions |
| 1 × 16 | Step tap Pick up beat of music *Gentle pulse raising* | | Bend deeper |
| 1 × 16 | Step tap and shoulder lifts *Mobilise shoulders* | Isolate shoulder lifts | |
| 1 × 16 | Step tap and shoulder rolls *Mobilise shoulders* | Isolate shoulder rolls | |
| 1 × 16 | Step tap and reach arms in front *Pulse raising and shoulder mobility* | Step tap without reach | |
| 1 × 16 | Step tap and reach arms over head | Keep arms to front | |
| 2 × 16 | Leg curls with arm pull backs *Knee mobility and pulse raise* | Place hands on hips | Bend deeper Increase reps |
| 1 × 16 | March in place *Pulse raising* Repeat plie squats pressing ball forward | | |
| 4 × 16 | Side squat right × 2 Side squat left × 2 Press ball forward *Pulse raise* Repeat | Place hands on hips | Bend deeper |
| 2 × 16 | Spine twists with ball *Spine mobility* | Without ball | |
| 2 × 16 | Step and knee lifts with arm pull downs *Hip mobility and pulse raise* | Place hands on hips Bicep curl arms | Travel forward × 4 Static × 4 Travel back × 4 Static × 4 Can add full turn on static lifts. 90 degree turn on each step |
| | Repeat from side squats if necessary | | |

*NB*: This warm up has been planned assuming the core ball and dumbbells are positioned in front of each participant.

| Table 12.4 | General preparatory (warm up) stretching for core ball class (Mixed ability) | | |
|---|---|---|---|
| **Timing** | **Exercise Description and Purpose** | **Alternative** *For more skilled* | **Progression** *For more skilled* |
| 1 × 32 | A. Side squat (2 R and 2 L) | Smaller bend | Deeper bend |
| 1 × 16 | B. Back lunges (right leg lead) | Smaller lunge | Combine with pectoral stretch |
| 10 secs | Into static *calf stretch* right | | |
| 10 secs | Static *quad stretch* right | Hold wall for balance | Can bend and straighten support knee whilst stretching |
| 10 secs | Static *hamstring stretch* right | Smaller bend at hip | Lift buttock higher on stretching leg |
| 1 × 32 1 × 16 | Repeat A and B (left lead) | | Combine calf stretch with trapezius stretch |
| 10 secs × 3 | Repeat stretches left leg | | |
| 1 × 32 10 secs 10 secs 10 secs | Step tap *Stretch triceps* R and L *Stretch pectorals* *Stretch trapezius* | Isolate stretches without leg movement | Triceps only if other stretches combined with lower body stretches. |
| 1 × 16 | Wide squats | Shallow bend | Deeper bend |
| 1 × 16 | Side bends *Spine mobility* | | |
| 10 secs | Oblique stretch | Reach up no side bend | Increase bend to side |
| 1 × 16 10 secs | Wide squats Into double adductor stretch | Single leg adductor stretch | Single leg adductor stretch with oblique stretch |
| 1 × 16 | D. Side lunges with lateral raise Pulse raising | Leave out arms | Deeper bend |
| 1 × 32 | Repeat C and D above | | |

*NB*: For specific progressions and adaptations for each stretch position refer to chapter XXXXXX

| Table 12.5 | Seated/Supine lying on ball MSE for core ball class (Mixed ability) | | |
|---|---|---|---|
| **Reps, Speed & Stick diagram** | **Exercise Description and Purpose** | **Adaptation (For less fit)** | **Progression (For more advanced)** |
| 1-1 × 16 | A. Leg extension (R + L) | Smaller raise | Increase reps |
| 1-1 × 16 | *Quads* | Less reps | Decrease speed |
| 2-2 × 16 | B. Dumbbell shoulder press *Deltoids, Triceps, upper trapezius* | Less reps Lighter resistance | Increase reps Increase resistance |
| | Repeat A and B Roll down to lying on ball | | |
| 2-2 × 16 | C. Abdominal curls (lying on ball) *Rectus Abdominus* | Floor lying Decrease reps | Add dumbbell resistance |
| 2-2 × 16 | D. Dumbbell chest press (lying on ball) *Pectorals, triceps, anterior deltoids* | Floor lying Decrease reps | Add 3-1 and 1-3 speed variation |
| | Repeat C and D Roll up to sitting on ball | | |
| 2-2 × 16 | E. Dumbbell Bicep curl *Biceps* | 1 × 12 | Increase resistance |
| 2-2 × 16 | F. Overhead Dumbbell Tricep press *Triceps* | 1 × 12 | Increase resistance |
| | Repeat E and F to superset | No repeat or rest between sets | |

| Table 12.6 | Prone lying on ball MSE for core ball class (Mixed ability) | | |
| --- | --- | --- | --- |
| **Reps, Speed & Stick diagram** | **Exercise Description and Purpose** | **Adaptation (For less fit)** | **Progression (For more advanced)** |
| 1-1 × 16 | A. Back extension | Smaller raise | Increase reps |
| | *Erector spinae* | Less reps | Decrease speed 2-2 |
| 2-2 × 16 | B. Prone flyes<br>*Trapezius* | Less reps<br>No resistance | Increase reps<br>Increase resistance |
| | Repeat A and B | | |
| 1-1 × 20<br>1-1 × 20 | C. Rear leg raises (R + L)<br>*Gluteus Maximus* | Floor lying<br>Decrease reps | Decrease speed 2-2 |
| 2-2 × 16 | D. Press ups<br>(knees on ball)<br>*Pectorals, Triceps, Anterior Deltoids* | More of body on ball<br>Decrease reps | Less of body on ball to increase core fixation. |
| | Repeat C and D | | |

| Table 12.7 | Floor lying MSE for core ball class ( Mixed ability) | | |
| --- | --- | --- | --- |
| **Reps, Speed & Stick diagram** | **Exercise Description and Purpose** | **Adaptation (For less fit)** | **Progression (For more advanced)** |
| 1 × 5 -10 | Abdominal Bridge<br>*Core stabilisers.* | Closer to ball | Further away from ball |
| 1-1 × 20 | Supine crook lying (on back with feet on ball)<br>A. Curl up<br>*Rectus abdominus* | 1 × 12-16<br>rest before next exercise | 1-1 × 8<br>2-2 × 8<br>3-1 × 4<br>1-3 × 4 |
| 1-1 × 20 | Supine crook lying<br>B. Twisting sit up<br>*Obliques* | 1 × 12-16<br>rest before next exercise | Decrease speed And bring opposite knee to each elbow |
| | Rest and repeat | | |
| 1-1 × 12 | Supine lying with heels on ball<br>*Bridge and ball roll* | Just abdominal bridge<br>Decrease repetitions | Increase repetitions |

| Table 12.8 | Post workout stretch – for core ball class (Mixed ability) | | |
|---|---|---|---|
| **Length of hold & Stick diagram** | **Exercise Description and Purpose** | **Alternative position & stick diagram** | **Progression & adaptation** |
| 30 secs develop R & L | Supine lying – hamstrings | Seated hamstrings | P – ease leg straighter A – Hold a towel around leg |
| 15 secs maintain R & L | Supine lying – gluteal stretch | Seated gluteal stretch | P – ease leg closer A – Keep leg on floor |
| 15 secs maintain R & L | Supine lying – oblique stretch | Seated oblique stretch | P – take legs closer to floor, hold longer A – Only a small bend |
| 30 seconds | Seated adductor stretch | Seated straddle/ wide leg position | P – ease knees down further A – Hands on floor behind back to assist upright sitting position. |
| 10 – 15 secs maintain R & L | Seated tricep stretch | Take arm across the front of the body (stretches posterior deltoid and little tricep) | P – use other arm behind back & link hands to increase stretch A – press from front |
| 15 secs maintain | Seated pectoral stretch | Standing if seated position uncomfortable for back | P- raise arms slightly higher A – place hands on floor behind back |
| 10 secs maintain | Seated trapezius stretch | Standing if seated position uncomfortable for back | P – wrap arms around body and drop head forward A – small round of upper back. |
| 15 secs | Standing calf stretch | Seated with legs out straight. Place right heel on top of left foot and use heel to draw toes of lower leg towards knee | P – use wall to lean further into stretch A – use wall for balance |
| 10 secs | Standing quad stretch | Use wall for balance | P - Tilt pelvis further forward |

*NB*: Stretches can be performed on ball after specific muscle work has ceased.

# REFERENCES AND RECOMMENDED READING

American College of Sports Medicine – *Guidelines for Exercise Testing and Prescription* (Lea and Febiger, 1991)

Bassey, E. and Fentam, P. – *Exercise. The facts* (Oxford University Press, 1981)

Bean, A. – *The Complete Guide to Sports Nutrition* (Second edition) (A & C Black, 1996)

Borg, G.V. – Psychophysical Basis of Perceived Exertion. *Medicine and Science in Sports and Exercise.* Journal 14 (5) (pp. 377–381)

Bursztyn, P. – *Physiology for Sports People. A user's guide to the body* (Manchester University Press, 1990)

Cullum, R. and Mowbray, L. – *The English YMCA Guide to Exercise to Music* (Pelham Books, 1995)

Devereux, G. – *Dynamic Yoga* (Thorsons, 1998)

Fostater, M. & Manuel, J. – *The Spiritual teachings of Yoga* (Hodder and Stoughton, 2002)

Fox, E. – *Sports Physiology* (Saunders College Publishing, 1984)

Gargrave, R., Lawrence, D. and Patrickson, J. – *Step Training Manual* (YMCA Fitness Industry Training, 1993)

Hazeldine, R. – *Fitness for Sport* (The Crowood Press, 1985)

Hine, J. – *Yang Tai Chi Chaun* (A & C Black, 1992)

Keighley, J. and Gargrave, R. – *Fitness Training Manual* (YMCA Fitness Industry Training, 1992)

Lawrence, D. – *The Complete Guide to Exercise in Water* (A & C Black, 1998)

McArdle, W., Katch, F. and Katch, V. – *Exercise Physiology* (Lea and Febiger, 1991)

McNeill Alexander, R. – *The Human Machine* (Natural History Museum Publications, 1992)

Mitchell, L. – *Simple Relaxation. The Mitchell Method for Easing Tension* (John Murray, 1987)

Norris, C. – *Abdominal Training* (A & C Black, 1997)

Norris, C. – *Flexibility, principles & Practice* (A & C Black, 1994)

Robinson, L., Fisher, H., Knox, J., Thompson G. – *The official Body Control Pilates Manual* (MacMillan, 2000)

Smith, H. (ed) – *Introduction to Human Movement* (Addison-Wesley, 1968)

Thompson, C. – *Manual of Structured Kinesiology* (Times Mirror/Mosby, 1985)

Woodham, A. – *Beating Stress at Work* (Health Education Authority, 1995)

# USEFUL ADDRESSES

## Pilates Teacher Training

**Body Control Pilates teacher training**
14, Neal's Yard,
London, WC2 9DP

**Modern Pilates Training**
Northern Fitness and Education
9a Cleasby Road,
Menston,
Ilkey
Leeds, LS29 6JE.

**Pilates Institute and Michael A King Ltd.**
Third floor, Wimbourne House,
151-155 New North Road,
London, N1 6TA.

## Yoga Teacher training

**Godfrey Devereux**
Dynamic Yoga teacher training
36, Stanbridge Road,
London. SW15 1DX

## Exercise to Music Teacher Training

(including step, studio resistance training, supple strength and core stability)

**YMCA Fitness Industry Training**
The Lesley Mowbray Suite,
111, Great Russell Street,
London, WC1B 3BR

## Music companies

**Solid Sound UK Ltd.**
PO Box 5978,
Laindon,
Basildon, Essex. SS15 4DX

**Pure Energy**
Music factory entertainment group
Hawthorne House,
Fitzwilliam street,
Parkgate,
Rotherham,
South Yorkshire, S62 6EP

**Fitness Professionals Ltd**
113, London Road,
London. E13 0DA.

# INDEX